It is ironic that one of the wealthiest and most successful nations on earth, the United States of America, has continued to struggle with the humanitarian concept that should be natural to us all: comprehensive, high quality, affordable health care for everyone. Yet we have the most expensive system of all nations, which performs poorly in contrast to other wealthy nations. Fortunately, John Geyman provides us with an explanation of how we arrived at this sorry state, and, more importantly, how we can use our national wealth to provide quality care for everyone, by adopting the policies of a well-designed, single payer system, sometimes referred to as an improved Medicare for All. In these difficult political times, we need to unify to show that we will support a national leadership that shows support for us, the people, by enacting and implementing such a system that takes care of all of us rather than promoting a perverse system designed to take care of the billionaires.

—Don McCanne, M.D., family physician, senior health policy fellow and past president of Physicians for a National Health Program (PNHP)

This essential primer details the origins and contours of the current disastrous state of American healthcare, the added peril posed by Donald Trump, and the salutary alternative that could save lives and money.

—David Himmelstein, M.D. and Steffie Woolhandler, M.D. are American primary care physicians and medical researchers. They are advocates for single-payer health insurance in the United States. Both were founding board members of Physicians for a National Health Program (PNHP).

GROWING COSTS OF U. S. HEALTH CARE

Corporate Power vs. Human Rights

Is Reform Finally Within Reach?

John Geyman, M.D.

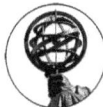

Copernicus Healthcare
Friday Harbor, Washington

Growing Costs of U.S. Health Care
Corporate Power vs. Human Rights
Is Reform Finally Within Reach?

John Geyman, M.D.
Copernicus Healthcare, Friday Harbor, WA

First Edition
Copyright ©2025 by John Geyman, M.D.
All rights reserved

Front cover photo:
    ID 137206551 © Dragan Andrii | Dreamstime.com
Back Cover photo:
    ID 280151820 © Puttachat Kumkrong | Dreamstime.com
Author photo by Anne Sheridan.

softcover: ISBN 978-1-938218-45-3
Library of Congress Control Number: 2025905065

Copernicus Healthcare
34 Oak Hill Drive
Friday Harbor, WA 98250

DEDICATION

To the many millions of Americans struggling to gain access to necessary health care in our failing health care system designed as it is to meet the needs of corporate interests, not those of us as patients. And to the hundreds of thousands of health care professionals trying to cope with a dysfunctional and bureaucratic system that takes their time away from serving patients. And to the growing army of citizen activists committed to health care reform. May this country find a way to finance health care that provides universal coverage for all residents and return medicine to its traditional ethic of service.

CONTENTS

PREFACE:... I

PART I: HOW DID WE GET HERE?.................................... III

Chapter 1: Reform Attempts of U. S. Health Care 1
Chapter 2: Barriers to Health Care Reform 11

PART II: TODAY'S HEALTH CARE "SYSTEM" 25

Chapter 3   How Corporate Privateering Has Disrupted
            U.S. Health Care 27

PART III: WHY THE U.S. "SYSTEM" NEEDS REFORM 41
Chapter 4: Increasing Privatization of Health Care.................. 43
Chapter 5: Loss of Patient Protections 59
Chapter 6: Declining Access to Affordable Health Care........... 69
Chapter 7: Abortion and Reproductive Rights.......................... 83
Chapter 8: Increased Bureaucracy, Corruption, Waste
            & Fraud.. 91
Chapter 9: Deregulation of Health Care 101
Chapter 10: Inadequate Oversight and Accountability.............. 111

PART IV: TOWARD A BRIGHT FUTURE WITH
            NATIONAL HEALTH INSURANCE.................... 123

Chapter 11: Current Crisis in U.S. Health Care 125
Chapter 12: Long Overdue for the U. S: National Health
            Insurance.. 139

Index 149
About the Author 165

TABLES AND FIGURES

Figure 1.1.   Growth of Physicians and Administrators, 1970-2019 5

Figure 1.2.   Medicare and Medicaid keep Private Insurers Afloat 5

Figure 1.3   Rise of the 1% and Fall of Bottom 50%, 1980-2016 6

Figure 1.4   Decline of Middle-Income Aggregate Wealth in the U. S.,
                1983-2016 6

Figure 1.5   Corporate Contributions to Influence Federal Elections
                after Citizens United 7

Figure 1.6   Who Does Congress Listen To? 8

Table 3.1   Corporate "Alliance" for Health Care Reform
                —The Big Four 33

Figure 3.1   Real GDP Recovery in the G7 Relative to Pre-Pandemic 35

Figure 4.1   Extent of For-Profit Ownership, 2016 46

Table 4.1   Comparative Features of Privatized and Public Medicare 47

Table 4.2   Quality of Care in VA versus Non-VA Hospitals 51

Figure 5.1   Percent of Adults Ages 50-64 with a Declinable Pre-Existing
                Condition 60

Figure 5.2   States Banning Abortion and Expansion of Medicaid 65

Figure 6.1   Total U.S. Health Spending and Medicaid Spending 72

Figure 7.1   States Where Abortion is Legal, Banned or Under Threat 86

Figure 9.1   The Green Wave of Dark Money 106

Figure 11.1   America's Health Care Divide
                —Health Systems Vary Across U.S. 133

Figure 11.2   Mirror, Mirror, A Portrait of the Failing U.S. Health
                System 2024, *The Commonwealth Fund* 133

Table 12.1   Value-Based Comparison of Four Alternatives 141

Table 12.2   Evidence-Based Comparison of Four Alternatives 141

Table 12.3   Winners and Losers Under National Health Insurance 145

ACKNOWLEDGEMENTS

As with my previous books, I am indebted to many for making this book possible. Thanks are especially due to many investigative journalists, health professionals, and others for their probing reports on our evolving, dysfunctional health care system. The work of many organizations has been useful in gathering evidence-based information on what is actually happening in U.S. health care, including the Kaiser Family Foundation, the Commonwealth Fund, the Center for National Health Program Studies, Public Citizen's Health Research Group, the Centers for Medicare and Medicaid Services, the U. S. Government Accountability Office, and the Congressional Budget Office.

WBC Design, an associate of Copernicus Healthcare, has once again done a great job from start to finish, including cover design and interior layout.

Most of all, I am grateful to my wife, Emily, for her helpful suggestions and encouragement throughout the process.

PREFACE

Since the Republican Congress and Trump administration failed to repeal and replace the Affordable Care Act (ACA) or ObamaCare, we have seen widespread confusion and anger among the public as to what is really going on in health care. As a result, most Americans are increasingly anxious about whether they can afford insurance and health care. Even those already covered by Medicare and Medicaid are worried about threatened cutbacks and increased costs as Congressional Republicans dedicate themselves to slashing "entitlement" funding to help pay down the $1.5 trillion deficit resulting from the 2017 passage of their tax bill. Fast forward to today and our embattled Trump presidency. After many Trump Executive Orders, we are waiting to see if we have a democracy after the initial chaos wears off.

In mid-October, 2017, President Trump issued an executive order intended to hasten the demise of ObamaCare. It called for government agencies to expand association health plans by allowing them to form groups across state lines, to expand the marketing of low-cost, barebones insurance for periods less than 12 months, and encourage wider use of health reimbursement accounts (HRAs) by employers for their employees. None of those directions improved access to care or addressed systemic problems of high health care costs. The federal government increasingly shifted the burden for health care to the states, including through block grants, giving them more flexibility (and less accountability) for their own programs and "saving" the government money. As columnist David Leonhardt observed:

> *TrumpCare has begun, not through legislation but through executive action . . . In doing so, it has both the short-term goal (have the federal government do less to help vulnerable citizens) and a long-term goal (sabotage ObamaCare, so that Congress can more easily repeal the law).* [1]

ObamaCare has been so undermined by past and ongoing actions of the Trump administration that we can no longer call the ACA ObamaCare. It is now TrumpCare, with Trump and Republicans in Congress owning it. The new recommendations brought forward by the Heritage Foundation's *2025 Report: A Conservative Promise* call for similar directions should Trump be re-elected president in 2024.

We have come to a place where the "Magic of the Marketplace" and neoliberalism have brought us to a confrontation between an authoritarian state and the common good.

The future of health care in the U.S. is dependent on the outcome of the battle between privatization, BIG MONEY and the corporate state versus a reformed system meeting the needs of our entire population. Back in 1812, Thomas Jefferson warned us about these circumstances.

Power always thinks it has a great Soul, and vast Views beyond the Comprehension of the Weak, and that is doing God's Service, when it is violating All his Laws. [2]

What end up as factual words from President Trump depends on future legal results. This book will deal with today's times in health care. We will see what happens.

—John Geyman, M.D.
Friday Harbor, WA,
June 1, 2025

References

1. Leonhardt, D. How to fight the new TrumpCare. *New York Times*, October 15, 2017.
2. Trump, D. J. as quoted by Cunningham, P W. A eulogy for the individual mandate. *The Washington Post*, December 21, 2017.

Part I

HOW DID WE GET HERE?

The process and outcomes of the 2024 elections in the United States, up and down the ballot, were indeed historic. At the presidential level, Donald J. Trump won by the barest of margins—winning the popular vote by just 49.8 percent versus his Democratic opponent, Kamala Harris at 48.3 percent. Outcomes in Congress were likewise close, with thin margins favoring Republicans.

Despite their importance, the growing costs of health care, together with limited access and related problems, had received little attention during the campaign. While Trump had said for years that he has "a plan" for health care, any details of what that means have remained obscure.

As we shall see shortly in this book, the long-term problems of U. S. health care continued without much change throughout his first term, 2017-2021. All of those goals fell by the wayside, so what might we expect with his second term? In the several weeks following the election, future directions for U. S. health care started to clarify as leaders were announced by incoming President Trump.

We are all aware of Trump's continued lies and lack of substance on policy issues. He has been upfront, however, on his overall goals after election this time, all intended to increase his political power:

- Bring independent agencies under presidential control,
- Revive the practice of "impounding funds,"
- Strip employment protections from tens of thousands of longtime civil servants,
- Purge officials from intelligence agencies, law enforcement, the State Department, and the Pentagon,
- and appoint lawyers who would bless his agenda as lawful.

With that backdrop, Trump's choice of leaders announced during the weeks after the election tells us more what lies ahead in health care.

- Robert F. Kennedy, Jr., as Secretary of Health and Human Services: vaccine skeptic and science denialist, to take over the large department with an annual budget over $1.7 trillion, 80,000 employees, major funder of U. S. health care. [1]
- Dr. Mehmet Oz, cardiac surgeon and TV personality, to head the Centers for Medicare and Medicaid Services (CMS) who will advance privatization of programs including Medicare Advantage. [2]

As discussions over how the Democrats lost the election consume the media, we are certainly at a new time of challenges to our democracy. The non-partisan Pew Research Center tells us we are in a new world of realignment news in a media ecosystem, with its disinformation having been a key factor leading to Trump's election. Now it is time to take a closer look at what brought U. S. health care to this uninhabitable place.

We can expect chaos along the way. As presidential historian Jon Meacham observed after the election:

> *Trump's concerted efforts to overthrow the November 2020 election very nearly succeeded—tangible proof that he is in fact ready to follow through on the authoritarian threats he so freely makes, I now see him as a genuine aberration in our history—a man whose contempt for constitutional democracy makes him a unique threat to our nation.*[3]

—Professor of History at Vanderbilt University

The business model of U.S. Health Care, as mediated through the profiteering private health insurance industry, is what we have inherited for reform.

This book will deal with these times in health care. We shall see what happens!

References:

1. Whyte, LE, Restuccia, A, Salama, V. Trump chooses RFK Jr. as health secretary. *Wall Street Journal*, November 15, 2024, p. A:1.
2. Diamond, D. RFK Jr. weighs major changes to how Medicare pays physicians.
3. Jon Meacham author of *And There was Light: Abraham Lincoln and the American Struggle*

Note:

In this book, the terms Medicare for All and single payer refer to National Health Insurance (NHI).

Chapter 1

Reform Attempts of U. S. Health Care

We're going to have insurance for everybody. People can expect to have great health care. It will be in a much-simplified form. Much less expensive and much better.[1]

—Donald Trump, before his inauguration.
The Washington Post, January 15, 2017.

Here is Trump in the above quote 8 years ago before his inauguration in 2017, vacuous as usual as a multimillionaire or billionaire, posturing as a pseudo-populist. He was seeming to support universal health care, but lying through his teeth as he has done regularly since running for president and in his first presidential term. With all that supposed dedication to universal health care, why did we not see progress toward health care reform in Trump's four years as president? As we all know so well, he has very little knowledge about policy in any area, changes his mind via tweets on a frequent, even daily basis, and appears to have no historical knowledge or principles of his own.

His above statement was as uninformed and incoherent as we see every day today on a wide range of subjects. Now he is fighting against any effort to broaden health care in the public interest, quite the opposite of his earlier declaration. His first administration, together with a Republican-controlled Congress, was committed to repealing the Affordable Care Act (ACA or ObamaCare) without any idea for a replacement plan, as it still is today.

This chapter has two major goals: to discuss past efforts to reform U. S. health care and achieve universal health care in this country; and (2) to review the more recent history of the surge of money into politics.

1

I.   *Historical Perspective*

As candidate for president in 1912 with the Progressive Party, Theodore Roosevelt made National Health Insurance (NHI) a platform plank. The trend over the previous 30 years had been to establish similar programs in many European countries, usually as sickness insurance, with Germany the leader in 1883.

Although T. R. lost the 1912 election, a social insurance committee of the American Medical Association actually adopted this resolution in 1917:

> *The time is present when the profession should study earnestly to solve the questions of medical care that will arise under various forms of social insurance. Blind opposition, indignant repudiation, bitter denunciation of these laws is worse than useless; it leads no-where and it leaves the profession in a position of helplessness as the rising tide of social development sweeps over it.*[2]

That resolution soon fell by the wayside as state chapters around the country denounced it, and the AMA has taken a reactionary position against national health insurance (NHI) ever since.

In the mid-1930s, President Franklin Delano Roosevelt considered including NHI in his New Deal agenda but backed off because of strong opposition from the AMA. Since then, the only real NHI proposal was made by President Harry Truman in 1946, but it again failed as opponents lobbied a Republican controlled Congress and played to the public's neo-Cold War fears of "socialism."[3]

Later efforts to reform U. S. health care fell way short of NHI. In the early 1970s, President Nixon offered his own "Play or Pay" proposal as an alternative to Ted Kennedy's single-payer plan. It would have required employers to either offer acceptable coverage to their employees or pay a tax that would finance their coverage from an insurance pool that would also cover the unemployed. Besieged as he was with the Vietnam War and Watergate, Nixon's proposal went through several iterations in Congress only to fail to gain sufficient support for coverage.[4]

The next major reform attempts in 1993-1994 included the Clinton Health Plan (CHP), a very complex proposal that combined employer mandates and spending controls. The Clinton plan attracted such intense controversy from most quarters that the 1,342 page bill never got out of committee to a vote in the House. It was strongly opposed by the insurance industry which fielded a national television campaign, "Harry and Louise", who sat around their kitchen table finding fault with the plan. Among several competing bills at the time, the single-payer plan proposed by Representative Jim McDermott (D-WA), the only one for NHI, had strong grassroots support, attracted the largest number of supporters in Congress, and was the only bill to pass out of committee. But it was soon lost in the shuffle and marginalized by the mainstream media as the war over the Clinton plan proceeded to its demise.

Passage of the ACA in 2010 was the signature domestic legislation of the Obama years. Democrats gave it strong support against an ongoing barrage of attacks by Republicans, who saw it as "a government takeover" when the opposite was true. Each health care industry profited immensely from the bill—insurers by gaining more enrollees and new streams of federal funding, hospitals by having more paying patients, and the drug industry by enlarging their markets and avoiding any price controls. Despite attacks from the GOP, some 24 million Americans gained coverage through becoming insured, especially through expansion of Medicaid in 31 states. Important patient protections were also in the bill, such as banning insurers from denying coverage for pre-existing conditions and allowing parents to keep their children on their coverage until age 26.

Republicans in Congress continued to vow to repeal and replace the bill at the earliest possible time, but when their time came after the 2016 elections, they failed repeatedly in that quest despite controlling the White House and both chambers of Congress. Republican legislators were divided among themselves. The far-right Freedom Caucus dug in over the need to cut Medicaid in the short and long term, further deregulate the insurance market to give consumers "more choice," shift control of health care back to the states through block grants and defund Planned Parenthood. Moderate Republicans pushed back, fearing re-election losses if more than 22 million people were to lose insurance if the ACA was repealed. The GOP was in a further quandary by having no replacement plan of its own, the opposition to any of their proposals by corporate stakeholders in the ACA, and continued strong public support for the ACA with little support for GOP proposals.

Since the 2016 elections, Republicans have been steadfast in sabotaging the ACA in any number of ways, hoping that it will implode on its own. Their supposed tax cut plan did repeal the ACA's individual mandate, causing heartburn among insurers. Many administrative initiatives have also been taken, including decreasing administrative funds promoting ACA's enrollment, cutting enrollment periods from 90 to 45 days, discontinuing cost-sharing reduction (CSR) payments to insurers, and proposed new rules by the Centers for Medicare and Medicaid (CMS) that would allow states to set up their own plans without responding to the ACA's constraints.

The revolving door was still in effect. As one example, Seema Verma helped to implement Medicaid "reform" in Indiana while Michael Pence was Governor. She was picked by Trump in his first term to head the Centers for Medicare and Medicaid (CMS). In that capacity she presided over an almost $1 trillion annual budget, planned to further privatize and cut back Medicare and Medicaid, and give states more latitude to avoid the ACA's restraints on insurer practices.

Taking a broad view, as our medical-industrial complex has expanded mightily since its inception in the 1980s, the growth of numbers of managers has grown exponentially during that time (Figure 1.1). Privatization of public programs has likewise expanded markedly, with the government keeping private health insurers afloat. (Figure 1.2).

Figure 1.1

GROWTH OF PHYSICIANS AND ADMINISTRATORS - 1970-2019

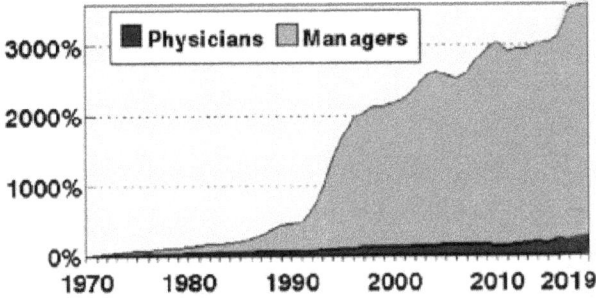

Source: Bureau of Labor Statistics; NCHS; and Himmelstein/Woolhandler analysis of CPS. Note - Managers shown as moving average of current year and 2 previous years

Figure 1.2

MEDICARE AND MEDICAID KEEP PRIVATE INSURERS AFLOAT

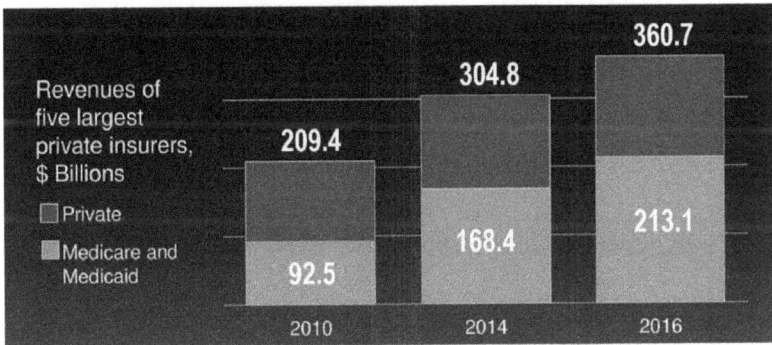

Source: *Health Affairs*; 36 (2):185, 2017

Other major developments were also taking place over the last 40 years, especially those that impacted negatively on societal issues. Two examples make the point: the remarkable increase in corporate CEO compensation in large corporate monopolies compared to worker compensation (Figure 1.3) and the decline of the middle class in the U. S. (Figure 1.4), which was likewise reflected in Europe.

Figure 1.3

RISE OF TOP 1% AND
FALL OF BOTTOM 50% 1980-2016

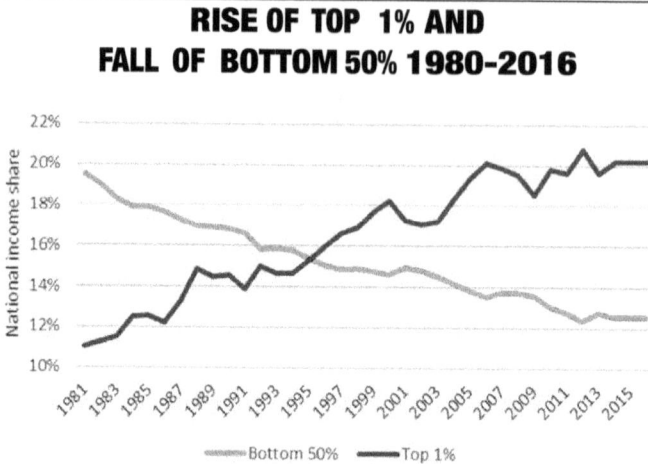

Source: Pew Research Center analysis of the Survey of Consumer Finances

Figure 1.4

DECLINE OF MIDDLE-INCOME AGGREGATE WEALTH
IN THE U.S., 1983-2016

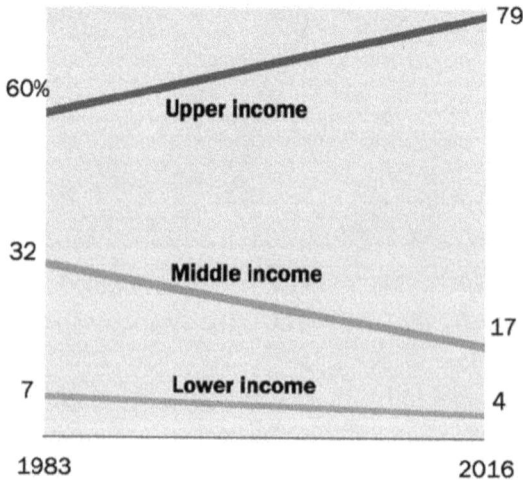

Source: Pew Research Center analysis of the Survey of Consumer Finances

II. *Surge of Money into Politics*

Fast forward to today— after many Executive Orders of the incoming Trump 2 administration, we have yet to see how our democracy will survive.

Figure 1.5 gives us graphic evidence that outside spending in federal elections since Citizens United in 2010 has skyrocketed over the last 15 years. [5] The Supreme Court declared that corporations have the same constitutional rights as real people do. In a follow-up ruling, the Supreme Court ruled that corporate spending on politics amounts to "speech" that is protected by the First Amendment. In its *Speech Now* case, it ruled that supposedly "independent" expenditures to help a political candidate cannot be regulated at all.

FIGURE 1.5

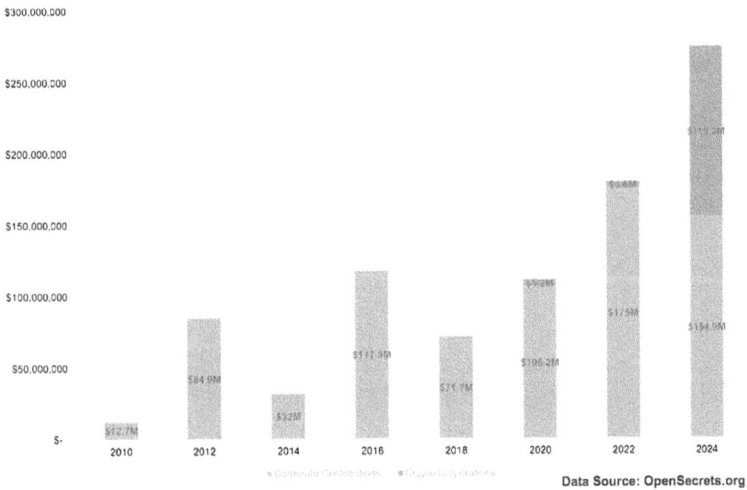

CORPORATE CONTRIBUTIONS TO INFLUENCE FEDERAL ELECTION AFTER *CITIZENS UNITED* HIGHLIGHTING CONTRIBUTIONS BY CRYPTO CORPORATIONS

Data Source: OpenSecrets.org

Source: Claypool, R. Crypto corporations dump $119 M. in attempt to buy 2024 elections. *Public Citizen News* 44/5, September/October, 2024, p. 6).

Much of the so-called "free speech" used during election campaigns has become altered by disinformation favoring election results in their originator's favor. The world's richest person, Elon Musk, bought Twitter with the explicit goal of molding it to his political interests. Soon thereafter, it was renamed X, which proceeded to spread disinformation throughout the 2024 election cycle. In Trump's election Silicon Valley found the president it wanted—supporting deregulation and an opponent of antitrust regulations.[6] Another example of weaponized information is Musk's America PAC, which funded a fraudulent "lottery" of $118 million favoring Trump during the 2024 election, with a plan to prepare for the 2026 midterms and any intermediate elections. [7]

If we think that legislators respond to the needs of their constituents more than to these contributions and the pressures from lobbyists, Figure 1.6 dispels that notion in both parties.

Figure 1.6

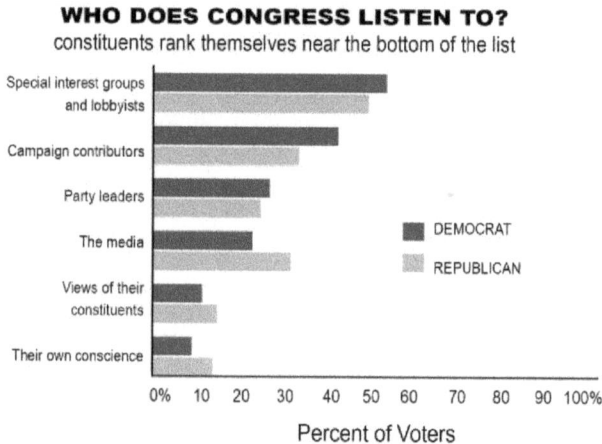

WHO DOES CONGRESS LISTEN TO?
constituents rank themselves near the bottom of the list

Source: Chris Cioffi, *Roll CAll*, Voters to Congress: Are you listening?,
March 17, 2021

As just one of many examples of corporate greed at work, General Motors announced a layoff of 2,500 workers. GM said that it had no choice, while its CEO compensation for 2024 was $27.8 million, the ratio of CEO-typical worker salary was more than 300:1, and the amount spent on stock buybacks was $6 billion. [8]

According to the Bureau of Labor Statistics, more than 135 million workers were laid off over the last three years. Stock buybacks, which were illegal until 1982, have become a common form of stock manipulation further enhancing 70 percent of corporate profits.[9]

The large amounts of corporate money spent during the 2024 elections certainly did make a difference for the GOP. As one example, it helped to displace Rep. Sherwood Brown from his Senate seat and preserve the GOP's advantage in the Senate while spending more than $130 million on the cryptocurrency sector. [10]

Trump's alliance with Elon Musk, the world's richest man, to lead the Department of Government Efficiency, is a classic example of corruption from the start. Lacking any experience with government efficiency and regulation, he already is the beneficiary of multiple government contracts, some under federal scrutiny. Lisa Gilbert, co-president of Public Citizen, knows what this means:

> *It is laughable to put the "ultimate corporate tycoon" in charge of a commission of government spending and regulations. This is the ultimate corruption. If anyone has any doubts whether the Trump government aims to serve regular people or the billionaires, they should now be resolved.* [11]

The very wealthy oppose government's role in helping ordinary Americans, according to polls of multimillionaires, people in the top 1 or 2 percent by wealth. Examples: 61 percent majority of the American public support national health insurance (NHI) financed by tax money vs. just 32 percent of the super wealthy; 68 percent of Americans believe that government must assure that nobody is without food, clothing and shelter vs. 43 percent of the multimillionaires.[12]

The continued problems of our health care system were among the leading issues facing the electorate in the November 2024 elections. Increasingly unaffordable health care costs, without containment on the horizon, were taking place as corporate giants gained speed through mega mergers. Our medical-industrial complex rolled on without significant reform as a paralyzed Congress allowed corporate stakeholders to continue to reap profits as a cash cow with no incentives to change.[13] Meanwhile, the urgency of health care reform as an overriding issue in the Democratic tool kit remained in a comparative sleeper position.

Concluding Comment

Given the above failures to enact a fix to runaway prices and costs of health care over more than a century in the U. S., it behooves us to examine the reasons for these shortfalls. We will take that on in the next chapter.

References:

1. President Trump before his inauguration. *The Washington Post*, January 15, 2017.
2. Burrow, JG. AMA: *Voice of American Medicine*. Baltimore. *Johns Hopkins Press*, 1963:144.
3. Thai, KV, Qiao, Y, McManus, SM. National health care reform failure: The political economy perspective. *J Health Hum Serv Adm*. Fall 1998: 21 (2): 236-259.
4. Iglehart, JK. Compromise seems unlikely on three major insurance plans. *National Journal Reports*. May 11, 1974; 6: 700-707.
5. Claypool, R. Crypto corporations dump $119 M. in attempt to buy 2024 elections. *Public Citizen News* 44/5, September/October, 2024, p. 6).
6. Angwin, J. The right's triumph over social media. *New York Times*, November 21, 2024, p. A:20.
7. Haake, S. Trump didn't win. Disinformation did. *The Progressive Populist*, December 1, 2024, p. 10.
8. Reich, R. GM, corporate greed, and the reason the Democrats lost the election.
9. Leopold, L. 135.9 million reasons why the working class is so angry. *The Progressive Populist,* November 15, 2024, p. 19.
10. Nerkar, S. $130 M. The total spent by the cryptocurrency sector to aid candidates who backed its agenda. *New York Times*, November 10, 2024, p. 2.
11. Johnson, J. 'Ultimate corporate corruption': Trump announces Musk-led department to gut regulations. *Common Dreams,* November 13, 2024.
12. Milbank, D. The Trump administration's days of blunder. *The Progressive Populist*, February 15, 2025, p. 21.,
13. Trump's decision to block U. S. aid heightens crises: Humanitarian impact. *New York Times*, February 2, 2025, p. A:1.

Chapter 2

Barriers To Health Care Reform

Market capitalism will have the same inefficient, exploitive outcome as Soviet Communism if the ownership of resources becomes concentrated in the hands of fewer and fewer large corporations, and if economic business decisions come to be made by those relatively few individuals who own and/or operate large, concentrated corporations.[1]

—Dr. Friedrich A Hayek, leading economist from the
last century and professor of social and moral sciences at the
University of Chicago, saw this coming as early as 1946.

In November 2024, President Trump won a second term in the White House, together with a bare majority in both houses of Congress. Growing problems in U. S. health care, including unaffordable costs, limited access and restricted access to care, place our country in last place among 10 high-income countries.[2] Health care reform will once again play a major role in the new administration. The stage could well be set for a more successful result *if* we can recognize and deal with the barriers to reform attempts over the last century that have blocked significant health care reform.

This chapter has three objectives: (1) to consider several myths that have been repeated so often as to become memes; (2) to describe the downsides of for-profit health care by corporations; and (3) to discuss some lessons that we can find helpful if we are to achieve successful future reforms.

I. Myths and memes

Many myths have evolved over the years and repeated so often as to become memes. Here are just three of the more important that still stand in the way of rational assessment of competing proposals.

1. The free market will fix our problems; competition works.

Despite Professor Hayek's prescient views of the future of health care markets, many economists have held the belief over many years that they work like other markets where competition can rein in prices and patients can shop for the best deal. In turn, most conservatives and those representing corporate stakeholders continue to promote this belief even though it has been fully discredited over the years for many reasons. Health care decision-making is not like shopping for the best deal on a new car. There is a knowledge gap between patients and health professionals, information is often unavailable, patients often don't know their needs, urgency of time is often a controlling factor as to who and where patients can access care, health insurers frequently restrict these choices, and consolidation of corporate providers invariably increases costs.

2. The private sector is more efficient than the public sector.

Market enthusiasts have long promoted the idea that the private sector is more efficient and provides more value to consumers than the public sector. Traditional Medicare as enacted in 1965 for everyone age 65 and older gives us an excellent example that rebuts this myth. Over more than the last 50 years, it has been run with a low overhead of about 2.5 percent and has proven to be a solid rock in a volatile health care marketplace. Compare this with private insurers that operate with administrative costs five times larger, restrict choice, cherry pick the market for favorable risk selection, impose higher deductibles and co-payments, disenroll sicker people, and withdraw from the market if it is not sufficiently profitable. [3]

3. *People with insurance overuse health care services.*

This assumption has underlain the conventional theory of health insurance based on the concept of "moral hazard", that holds that patients' behavior changes when they become insured, to the point that they abuse the system. The trend toward "consumer driven health care" (CDHC) in recent decades has been based on this premise, assuming that imprudent choices can be avoided when patients are more financially responsible for their decisions and have "more skin in the game." Policies have therefore been adopted throughout our system that require more cost-sharing by patients with the goal of reining in health care costs.

Though this myth persists today, experience over the last 30 years has shown the failure of this approach to contain health care costs. Instead, more cost-sharing with patients leads many to forgo or delay necessary care, resulting in higher costs down the road and worse outcomes. We have also yet to admit that the purpose of higher deductibles is not to help patients but to decrease spending by insurers, employers, and government plans.[4]

II.   *Health Care by Corporations*

Corporatization and growth of for-profit health care has been the dominant trend in the U. S. over the last four decades. Corporate hospital chains were established within a few years after the enactment of Medicare and Medicaid in 1965. As the profits of investor-owned facilities and services grew rapidly, Wall Street became closely involved. Between 1965 and 1990, their corporate profits grew by more than 100 times, a pace almost 20 times greater than profits for all U. S. corporations. [5]

As Paul Starr, professor of sociology and public affairs at Princeton University, noted as early as 1982:

> *The rise of a corporate ethos in medical care is already one of the most significant consequences of the changing structure of medical care. It permeates voluntary hospitals, government agencies, and academic thought as well as profit-making medical care organizations. Those who talked about "health care planning" in the 1970s now talk about "health care marketing." Everywhere one sees the growth of a kind of marketing mentality in health care. And, indeed, business school graduates are displacing graduates of public health schools, hospital administrators, and even doctors in the top echelons of medical care organizations. The organizational culture of medicine used to be dominated by the ideals of professionalism and voluntarism, which softened the underlying acquisitive activity. The restraint exercised by those ideals grew weaker. The "health center" of one era is the "profit center" of the next.* [6]

Some readers may be surprised how extensive for-profit ownership had become by 2016 across our health care system: specialty hospitals (37 percent), hospice (63 percent), nursing homes (65 percent), home care (76 percent), dialysis (90 percent), Surgi-Centers (95 percent), and free-standing laboratory and imaging centers (100 percent).[7]

1. *Medical-industrial complex, with corporate economic and political power allied with Wall Street, opposes reform.*

In 1980, the late Dr. Arnold Relman, internist and former editor of *The New England Journal of Medicine*, coined the term "medical-industrial complex." He did so in describing the emergence of a new for-profit health care industry ranging from proprietary hospitals and nursing homes to diagnostic services, medical devices, hemodialysis, and the pharmaceutical and insurance industries. He gave us this warning 38 years ago:

> *This new "medical-industrial complex" may be more efficient than its not-for-profit competition, but it creates the problems of overuse and fragmentation of services, over emphasis on technology, and "cream skimming," and it may also exercise undue influence on national health policy. Closer attention from the public and the profession, and careful study are necessary to ensure that the "medical-industrial complex" puts the interests of the public before those of its stockholders.* [8]

2. Health care as a commodity, not a service

A sea change has occurred over the last four decades in this country which has taken the medical profession and health care from a cottage industry to a complex industry largely driven by business goals of profitability and financial bottom lines that are increasingly driven by the needs of investors. Health care has been reduced to a commodity for sale on an open market that is mostly controlled by ever-larger corporations. Almost two-thirds of physicians today are employees of these organizations, especially hospital systems with their affiliated ambulatory care facilities. As employees, they are subject to their employers' drive to increase their revenues.

3. Health care as a large part of the economy

The health care industry, as 20% of the U. S. economy, has become the single largest part of our economy. More than one-third of the nation's job growth since the recession hit in late 2007 has been in the health sector, the single biggest sector for job growth. As the system has become more complex and fragmented, it has become administratively top-heavy, with 16 other workers for every physician. One half of these are in administrative and other non-clinical roles, especially involving data entry and other aspects related to billing and reimbursement. [9]

4.   *Privatization of public programs, such as Medicare and Medicaid.*

This is another feature of this new environment. We have evolved a system of corporate welfare for the insurance, hospital, pharmaceutical and other industries that feeds on public programs at taxpayer expense. Two-thirds of U. S. health care costs are now paid for by the government—with our taxes. [10]

III.   *Takeaway Lessons from Failed Health Care Reform*

What can we learn from the battles over health care reform, particularly since the Clinton effort in the 1990s and the ACA in 2008-2010? There are definite parallels with today's battles and here are eight obvious takeaway lessons that we need to learn if we are to be successful in future reform efforts.

1.   *Previous reform attempts have been hijacked by corporate stakeholders*

Taking the ACA as an example, the interests of private insurers, hospitals, drug and medical device industries, organized medicine, and other stakeholders in our market-based system took precedence over the needs of patients for broad access to affordable, quality health care. The political process that led up to passage of the ACA involving the corporate alliance of the Big Four—the insurance industry, PhRMA, the hospital industry, and organized medicine—was described in my 2010 book, *Hijacked: The Road to Single Payer in the Aftermath of Stolen Health Care Reform.*[11] Bob Herbert, well known Op-Ed columnist for the *New York Times*, was spot on with this observation:

> *The drug companies, the insurance industry and the rest of the corporate high-rollers have their tentacles all over this so-called reform effort, squeezing it for all its worth. Meanwhile, the public—struggling with the worst*

economic downturn since the 1930s—is looking on with
great anxiety and confusion. If the drug companies and the
insurance industry are smiling, it can only mean that the
public interest is being left behind. [12]

Lobbying and influence peddling in the Beltway was rampant
as the ACA was being framed and crafted. Based on ideology
and political forces, there was never any likelihood that the new
marketplace could bring the needed reforms. It was a given that what
was spent on lobbying would bring far more revenue than its costs.
Robert Field, professor of law and of health policy and management
at Drexel University, observed:

> *The ACA set the stage for a financial boon for the*
> *health care industry in numerous ways. It enables millions*
> *of new customers to purchase individual policies. It permits*
> *Medicaid programs in many states to retain more managed*
> *care companies to administer benefits.*
> *It helps hospitals and many physicians to realize*
> *increased revenues by giving more of their patients access to*
> *the financial resources needed to pay for care. And, over time,*
> *countless other businesses will emerge and thrive under the*
> *ACA's government-created structure as the ingenuity of the*
> *private sector finds ways to thrive off its new public base.* [13]

2. *You can't contain costs by permitting for-profit health care industries to pursue their business ethic in a deregulated market.*

As one could have expected from long experience in this
country, markets have completely failed to rein in prices and costs of
health care. Quite the opposite as they have continued to escalate
for hospitals, physicians, drug and medical device manufacturers
and other parts of our system. One venture capitalist promoting

investment opportunities for private exchanges under the ACA saw the likelihood to "turn chaos into gold."[14] That is exactly what happened as health care stocks soared by almost 40 percent in 2013, the highest of any sector in the S & P 500.[15]

3.   *You can't reform the delivery system without reforming the financing system.*

The U. S. keeps missing the boat in trying to contain health care costs within a largely for-profit multi-payer financing system. Our attempts to reform the delivery system so as to cover more people at more affordable costs proves to be futile every time it is tried. In the aftermath of the ACA's enactment eight years ago, the private health insurance industry has become even more complex and intrusive as it continues to profit from new subsidized markets. Insurers keep trying to avoid sicker, costlier patients and gaming the system to maximize their profits and keep their shareholders happy.

In true health care reform, our goal should be to provide universal access for our entire population to affordable, quality care without discrimination against the sick, those with pre-existing conditions, the poor, or the unemployed. Dr. Samuel Metz, adjunct associate professor of anesthesiology at Oregon Health and Science University in Portland, offers these three rules to achieve financing reform, all based on the solid experience over many years in advanced countries around the world that have transparent, publicly accountable, not-for-profit financing systems:

1.   *If you want comprehensive care for more people for less money, reform the financing system.*
2.   *If you want a dramatic reduction in costs without compromising quality, reform the delivery system.*
3.   *If you want Rule # 2 to work, you must first apply Rule #1.*[16]

4. *In order to achieve the most efficient health insurance coverage, we need to have the largest possible risk pool.*

The larger and more diverse the risk pool, the more effective insurance can be in having healthier people share the costs of sicker people and keeping costs down. We know that 20 percent of the population accounts for 80 percent of all health care spending, while 5 percent of the population uses almost one-half of total spending. [17] As long as we have a large private insurance industry with some 1,300 insurers trying to avoid sicker patients, with millions of younger, healthier people choosing to be uninsured, we will have segmented risk pools that prevent efficiencies of a large risk pool. As other advanced countries have found years ago, sharing risk across their whole populations is the only way to provide universal coverage at affordable costs to patients, families, and taxpayers.

5. *We can no longer afford to keep bailing out a failed private health insurance industry.*

The multi-payer health insurance industry stands in the way of universal coverage, is obsolete, and provides insufficient value to be continuously bailed out by government and taxpayers. The industry has had a long run since the 1960s, when it adopted medical underwriting practices to avoid sicker people with the goal of increased profits. Today it is antithetical to reform as it games a subsidized financing system for higher revenues for its CEOs and shareholders on the backs of patients and taxpayers.

The government has been more than friendly to the industry for many years through such perks as long-standing tax exemptions for employer-sponsored insurance and overpayments to Medicare Advantage plans. The ACA increased these subsidies in more ways, including passing along cost-sharing reduction (CSR) payments, new "risk corridor" payments to protect insurers from losses, and expansion of private Medicare and Medicaid plans.

Under the ACA, insurers have still found ways to game the system for higher profits by such means as high-cost sharing, inadequate provider networks, denial of services, restrictive drug formularies, manipulation of risk scores to get higher Medicare payments, marketing short-term plans lasting less than one year as a way to avoid the ACA's requirements, and deceptive marketing practices. Even while continuing to receive large subsidies from the government, the industry consumes 15 to 20 percent of the health care dollar in bureaucracy, administrative overhead, and profits as it retains a top position on Wall Street's S & P 500.

The cost of private health insurance has become prohibitive for much of the population, even as its coverage becomes skinnier all the time. Insurers had factored in the loss of CSR subsidies, with large premium increases for 2018—116 percent in Arizona and more than 50 percent in other states. Insurers are pushing to offer barebones policies, and we have an epidemic of *under-insurance*. Aetna, the nation's third largest insurer, scaled back its coverage even after its second-quarter 2017 revenue jumped by 52 percent. [18] Mark Bertolini, Aetna's CEO, recently acknowledged that the ACA's exchanges are in a "death spiral." [19] More insurers are leaving markets, with about one-half of U. S. counties having only one insurer this year, while we can expect to see a growing number of bare counties without any insurers. Wendell Potter, former industry insider, sums up the future of the industry this way:

> Folks, we are guilty of magical thinking. We've fallen for insurers' deception and misdirection, hook, line, and sinker. And many of us can't be persuaded that we are being duped. Meanwhile, the shareholders of the big for-profits are laughing all the way to the bank. Every single day. [20]

6. Access to buying health insurance is not coverage if you can't afford it.

After the continued failures of the Republican-controlled Congress to repeal and replace the ACA, together with their inability to come up with any coherent replacement plan, the GOP has brought forward the vague and deceptive concept that "everyone should have the opportunity to buy health insurance if they so choose." This would be a fraudulent policy of "universal access," without any regard to affordability or quality of that coverage. During his nomination hearing before the Senate, Dr. Tom Price said:

> *I believe that every single American has access to the highest quality care and coverage that is possible.* [21]

This flawed concept is ludicrous and will go nowhere, as it completely fails to recognize that the cost of insurance and care for a typical family of four with employer-sponsored insurance is now about $28,000 a year (almost one-half of median household income). Universal access means nothing if people cannot afford insurance and care. As a result, many millions of people forgo or delay necessary care because of costs and end up with worse outcomes if and when they finally do get care.

7. We need a larger, not smaller, role of government to reform health care.

The obvious failure of market-based policies and deregulation to contain health care costs and make them affordable for Americans over these many years calls for a larger role of government if we are ever to achieve real universal access to health care in this country. It is beyond time to acknowledge that the neoconservative policies of past, recent, and current administrations have not worked. Corporate interests in the medical-industrial complex stand in the way of universal access as they continue on their profit-taking binge with little public accountability. Today's market-based system leaves an ever-larger part of the population without needed care and is unsustainable. We have yet to accept the necessity of government to assure that the public interest is being met. As Jacob Hacker, PhD, professor of political science at Yale University, recently observed:

> *The difference between the United States and other countries isn't the role of insurance; it's the role of government. More specifically, it's the way in which those who benefit from America's dysfunctional market have mobilized to use government to protect their earnings and profits . . . But in every other rich country, the government not only provides*

coverage to all citizens; it also provides strong counter pressure to those who seek to use their inherent market power to raise prices or deliver lucrative but unnecessary services . . . [22]

8. *Failed health care reform exposes our loss of the democratic process.*

The Trump administration is clearly bent on dismantling our democratic institutions, battling against the norms of judicial process, and fighting against the free press in an increasingly dictatorial approach to governance. As David Frum has said in his 2018 book, *Trumpocracy: The Corruption of the American Republic*:

> As President Trump is cruel, vengeful, egoistic, ignorant, lazy, avaricious and treacherous, so we must be kind, forgiving, responsible, informed, hardworking, generous, and patriotic. As Trump's enablers are careless, cynical, shortsighted, morally obtuse, and rancorous, so Trump's opponents must be thoughtful, idealistic, wise, morally sensitive, and conciliatory. [23]

Concluding Comment

Noam Chomsky, Ph.D., professor emeritus of linguistics and philosophy at the Massachusetts Institute of Technology and author of the 2016 book, *Who Rules the World?*, brings this perspective to our circumstances and political challenges today:

> Beginning in the 1970s, partly because of the economic crisis that erupted in the early years of that decade and the decline in the rate of profit, but also partly because of the view that democracy had become too widespread, an enormous, concentrated, coordinated business offensive was begun to try to beat back the egalitarian efforts of the post-war era, which only intensified as time went on. The economy itself shifted to financialization. Financial institutions expanded enormously. By 2007 right before the crash for which they had considerable responsibility, financial institutions accounted for a stunning 40 percent

of corporate profit. A vicious cycle between concentrated capital and politics accelerated, while increasingly wealth concentrated in the financial sector. Politicians, faced with the rising cost of campaigns, were driven ever deeper into the pockets of wealthy backers. And politicians rewarded them by pushing policies favorable to Wall Street and other powerful business interests. Throughout this period, we have a renewed form of class warfare directed by the business class against the working people and the poor, along with a conscious attempt to roll back the gains of previous decades. [24]

Professor Chomsky's astute observation leads us directly into the next chapter, where we will consider how health policy in this country is bought and sold by the highest bidders.

References:

1.   Hayek, FA. The use of knowledge in society. *Am Econ Rev* 35: 519-530, 1946.
2.   Gunja, MZ et al. U. S. seniors experience worst cost barriers to care. *Health Justice Monitor*, December 4, 2014.
3.   Terhune, C. Health companies race to catch UnitedHealth as Amazon laces up. *Kaiser Health News*, November 3, 2017.
4   McCanne, D. Comment in quote-of-the-day on the November 2016 NBER Working Paper 22802, *National Bureau of Economic Research,* Cambridge, MA, November 7, 2016.
5.   U. S. Department of Commerce. The National Income and Products Accounts of the United States, 192901082L Statistical Tables, Table 6.21B. Washington, DC : U.S. Department of Commerce.
6.   Starr, P. *The Social Transformation of American Medicine.* New York. *Basic Books*, 1982, p. 448.
7.   Commerce Department, Service Annual Survey 2016 or most recent available date for share of establishments.
8.   Relman, AS. The new medical-industrial complex. *N Engl J Med* 303: 963-970, 1980.
9.   Terhune, C. Health care in America: An employment bonanza and a run- away-cost crisis. *Kaiser Health News,* April 24, 2017.
10. Himmelstein, DU, Woolhandler, S. The current and projected taxpayer shares of U. S. health costs. *Amer J Public Health online,* January 21, 2016.

11. Geyman, JP. Hijacked: The Road to Single Payer in the Aftermath of Stolen Health Care Reform. Friday Harbor, WA. *Copernicus Healthcare*, 2010, pp. 7-36.
12. Herbert, B. This is reform? *New York Times*, August 17, 2009.
13. Field, RI. Mother of Invention: How the Government Created "Free-Market" Health Care. New York. *Oxford University Press*, 2014, pp. 220-221.
14. Suennen, L. Here come the exchanges ... And the opportunity to turn chaos into gold. *Venture Valkyrie*, October 6, 2013.
15. Soltas, E. Nobody should get rich off Obamacare. *Bloomberg View*, December 3, 2013.
16. Metz, S. Reducing health care costs: delivery vs. financing approaches. Health Care Disconnects, November 12, 2013 (available at www.copernicus-healthcare.org)
17. National Institute for Health Care Management. A comparatively small number of sick people account for most health care spending. August 2, 2012.
18. Murphy, T. Aetna trumps 2Q expectations after scaling back ACA coverage. *ABC News*, August 3, 2017.
19. Johnson, C. Aetna chief executive says Obamacare is in a 'death spiral.' *The Washington Post*, February 15, 2017.
20. Potter, W. It's way past time for us to stop deluding ourselves about private health insurers. *The Progressive Populist*, September 1, 2016, p. 20.
21. Price, T, as quoted in Access to buying insurance is not health coverage. *Common Dreams*, January 19, 2017.
22. Hacker, JB. Why an open market won't repair American health care. *New York Times*, April 4, 2017.
23. Frum, D. Trumpocracy: *The Corruption of the American Republic*. New York. *HarperCollins*, 2018, p. 235.
24. Chomsky, N. As quoted by Polychroniou, CJ. Socialism for the rich, capitalism for the poor: An interview with Noam Chomsky. *Truthout*, December 16, 2016.

PART II

HOW DID WE GET TO TODAY'S HEALTH CARE "SYSTEM?"

Oh, what a tangled web we weave when first we practice to deceive.

—Sir Walter Scott

Coming to today's world, this expert in American politics sees these remarkable challenges before us as we work toward health care reform.

To my mind, there is no moral justification for electing Trump, although I think I understand why people voted for him. At the most basic level, they voted for him because for many decades they have not benefited from the fruits of their hard work. The median wage of the bottom 90 percent buys less today than it did 40 years ago. For decades, most of the gains have gone to the top. Grotesque inequalities of income, wealth, opportunity, and power have caused most Americans to feel angry, surly, cynical, and ready to take a wrecking ball to the whole system. But Trump's wrecking ball will only hurt most Americans and further enrich oligarchs like himself. We must help people understand this. [1]

—Reich, R. How to hope in a near-hopeless time? Thoughts on our horrendous loss of two weeks ago. robertreich@substack.com

Chapter 3

How Corporate Privateering
Has Disrupted U.S. Health Care

This is not a new problem, as TR found more than 100 years ago and as FDR noted in his famous re-election speech in 1936:

> *Moneyed interests had begun to think of the Government of the United States as a mere appendage to their own affairs. We know that government by organized money is as dangerous as Government by organized mob.* [1]

But today, arguably, this problem is the worst it has ever been and now threatens the survival of our supposed democracy.

This chapter has four goals: (1) to describe PhRMA, the pharmaceutical industry's trade group, as a poster child for this problem; (2) to consider how health policy and health care reform were subverted in the run-up to the ACA a decade ago; and (3) to briefly consider major legislation during the Biden years. and (4) to consider likely directions for Trump's second term.

I. PhRMA as the Poster Child for Profiteering and Corruption

Together with another trade group, the Biotechnology Innovation Organization, PhRMA (The Pharmaceutical Research and Manufacturers of America) set a new record for lobbying the federal government in 2017—almost $35 million. They were trying to protect themselves from any crackdown on drug pricing as well as any adverse impacts from the tax overhaul bill. PhRMA and its leading drug manufacturers have spent $1.8 billion on lobbying the federal government since 1999, according to the Center for Responsive Politics. These funds are carefully targeted to lawmakers, their staffers and regulators involving legislation either favorable or problematic to their interests. Daniel Auble, who tracks lobbying activity for the Center for Responsive Politics, had this to say after some 1,500 lobbyists swarmed Capitol Hill promoting passage of the 21st Century Cures Act in 2016: [2]

> *[This Act] is emblematic of the way laws get passed in Washington today: money is power, and no sector has more of both than the pharmaceutical industry.* [2]

In their ongoing attempts to retain their ability to set drug prices and avoid price controls, drug makers give money widely trying to defend their practices and gain friends and influence. As examples, PhRMA paid $14.3 million to think tanks, disease advocacy groups and universities in 2015,[3] while Pfizer gave $1 million to help finance Trump's inauguration.

The ties between the pharmaceutical industry and the federal government have been deepening for years, including through revolving doors *in both directions*—to and from Congress and the Department of Health and Human Services (DHHS). Almost 340 former congressional staffers now work for drug companies or their lobbying firms, according to Legistorm, a nonpartisan congressional research company. Those who go from drug companies to staff jobs on Capitol Hill often are able to maintain their drug industry pensions and stock, according to *Kaiser Health News*. [4]

Conflicts of interest are common within the revolving doors between industry, K street, and the government. Consider these examples:

- Dr. Tom Price (R-GA), while chairing the House Budget Committee, sitting on the House Ways and Means Committee, and with a history of contacting the FDA on behalf of industry donors, invested in a sweetheart deal in a new drug targeting the U. S. market by a tiny biotech firm Innate Immunotherapeutics. That investment went up by 400%. House financial disclosures require reporting of ranges of value, not specific amounts. As we know, he was Trump's first nominee to head DHHS, but was forced to resign as Secretary after disclosure of his use of private charter flights costing taxpayers more than $400,000.

- Alex Azar, Trump's second appointee to head DHHS, pocketed almost $2 million in compensation during his final year as president of drug giant Eli Lilly's U. S. operations, plus another $1.6 million in severance pay and as much as $1 million from sale of his Eli Lilly stock. During his tenure at Lilly, he presided over enormous price increases of Humalog insulin, which more than doubled between 2011 and 2016. [5] While at Lilly in 2009, he also helped to manage the fallout when Lilly paid a criminal fine of more than half a billion dollars to settle accusations that it had promoted Zyprexa, an anti-psychotic drug, for uses not approved by the FDA. [6]

PhRMA also targets state legislators with its lobbying efforts. A recent example is the industry's flooding the Louisiana state legislature with two lobbyists for every legislator to avoid passage of a bill that would require sales reps promoting medicines at physicians' offices to also reveal their prices. [7] PhRMA also gives big money to national political groups financing presidential, congressional, and state candidates, as well as patient advocacy groups for certain diseases. [8]

Price gouging is rampant throughout the drug industry, as well as in most other parts of the health care industry. The drug industry typically defends large price increases as required to offset its costs of bringing new drugs to market, which on its face is disingenuous. The industry wildly exaggerates the costs of bringing a new drug to market, with most of its claimed R & D costs being marketing and non-rigorous trials conducted by drug companies themselves. They continue to lobby for accelerated approval of new drugs by the FDA with lesser evidence for efficacy.

These examples of price gouging in health care have generated growing public outrage:

- Prices charged by U. S. manufacturers of COVID-19 vaccines exceeded production costs by more than 10-fold or more. [9]
- Early in the pandemic, Amazon hiked its prices for essential safety items, such as face masks and hand sanitizer, by up to 1,000 percent during a time of bidding wars. [10]
- By the end of the first pandemic year, the combined net worth of the richest Americans totaled $4 trillion, more than four times the price tag of the economic relief package being debated in Congress. [11]
- The costs of insulin have increased by 6-fold over the last 20 years, rendering this life-saving drug unavailable to many lower-income diabetic patients who cannot afford its monthly costs that can reach up to $1,200. [12]
- The costs of hospitals spread rapidly across the country, with the most expensive hospitals jacking up their charges by as much as 18 times costs. [13]
- With 70% of U. S. nursing homes for-profit, their emphasis is profiteering at the expense of adequate nursing staff and quality of care. [14]
- Revenue growth of major health insurers over the previous 10 years grew by 500% for privatized Medicare Advantage and Medicaid. [15]

In his January 2017 State of the Union address to Congress, President Trump called reducing prescription drug prices one of his "greatest priorities," adding that "prices will come down." This was almost certainly just another lie and broken promise, not because of the enormous political power of PhRMA, but also because of the opposition of Alex Azar as head of DHHS to negotiated drug prices by Medicare, as the VA has done for many years, effectively reducing the prices of prescription drugs by about 42 percent. Despite passionate calls for action by hospitals, physicians, insurers, and patients, there was little consensus about how to solve the problem and continued inaction in Congress.

We can see how the pharmaceutical industry is a good example of how corporate money and lobbying infiltrate government and dominate politics against the public interest. As a result, we have lost much of our supposed democratic process. As Wendell Potter and Nick Penniman say in their new book, *Nation on the Take: How Big Money Corrupts Our Democracy and What We Can Do About It*:

> *Our grand 240-year-old project of self-government has been derailed, replaced by a coin-operated system that mainly favors those who can pay to play.* [16]

II. How Outside Money Corrupted the ACA: 2008-2010

The Big Four—insurance industry, PhRMA, hospital industry, and the AMA— were the major players in the intense debate leading up to the passage of the ACA in 2010, but they were not the only ones. There were also many other players in the medical-industrial complex, ranging from the medical device and equipment industries to nursing homes and information technology. All wanted a seat at the table as competing bills moved forward in Congress. General Electric, as one example, then the 12th largest corporation in the world, had a big market share for imaging equipment and information technology. At that time, there were some 3,300 lobbyists in Washington D.C. spending $1.4 million a day lobbying for the special interests of these groups. [17]

These players were both defending their turfs and trying to expand their share of an expanded revenue pie to come under the guise of supporting reform. There was a blame game going on among these corporate interests as to who was responsible for the continued soaring costs of health care. As examples, insurers pointed to overcharging by hospitals, drug companies and physicians that left them no choice but to raise their premiums. Hospitals blamed physicians demanding higher payments as well as their rising burden of care for the uninsured and low reimbursement from Medicare and Medicaid.

There were conflicting interests and goals not only between these major players, but also within each group.

For example the hospital industry. The hospital industry was divided against itself, such as by divisions between urban and rural hospitals and between general and specialty hospitals.

Along the way in this contentious debate, there was some concern whether these corporate interests could forge a consensus. Finally voluntary, unenforceable pledges were made by the Big Four, which was soon labeled a "corporate alliance." Table 3.1 summarizes the pledges, agendas, tactics, and likely rewards for the Big Four stakeholders. [18] It is important to realize, however, that the public interest was left out of these negotiations, and that the revenues being sought by corporate stakeholders would become our costs as patients and taxpayers.

Three examples, all from the hospital and insurance industries, illustrate the subtle ways whereby health care industries can maximize their profits without much public awareness:

- Cumulative hospital mergers between 2000 and 2020 led to higher market-power price increases. [19]
- The long-term use of pharmacy-benefit managers by insurers in re-negotiating prices of drugs have led to marked increases in the costs of drugs distributed by hospitals. [20]
- Eight of the largest U. S. health insurers, with more than two-thirds of the privatized Medicare Advantage market, up coded their bills by at least $12 billion in overpayments in 2020. [21]

Over the years, it has become clear that the only way that corporate players could come to consensus would be if their investors would win. Indeed, Wall Street followed these negotiations closely, since the health care industry accounted for one-sixth of our economy. The insurance industry opposed the public option all along. When the Obama administration signaled its willingness to consider alternatives to a public plan, health insurer stocks were pushed higher despite a triple-digit loss in the broader markets. Trading in UnitedHealth and WellPoint jumped by about three-fold as investors placed calls and puts. [22]

Table 3.1

CORPORATE "ALLIANCE" FOR HEALTH CARE REFORM - THE BIG FOUR

Insurance Industry

Pledge	Abandon pre-existing conditions as an underwriting principle
	Accept all applicants
	Stop charging women higher premiums than men
Agenda	Grow private and public insurance markets by up to 50 million enrollees
Tactics	Oppose controls or caps on premium rates
	Oppose the public option
	Lobby for low standards for insurance coverage and low MLRs
	Fight against cuts of overpayments for Medicare Advantage plans
Rewards	Larger private and public markets
	Higher profits and returns to shareholders
	Preempt increased regulation by government

PhRMA

Pledge	$80 billion over 10 years toward costs of health care reform
Agenda	Expand private and public markets
	Avoid price controls and competition from importation of drugs from other countries
	Gain maximal patent protection for biotech drugs
Tactics	With assurance from White House agreement that government would not negotiate drug prices or import drugs from abroad, lobbied jointly with Families USA in support of health care reform as represented by bills in Congress
Rewards	Expanded private and public markets
	Higher profits and returns to shareholders
	Avoid increased regulation by government

Hospital Industry

Pledge	$155 billion over 10 years in reduced hospital charges
Agenda	Growth in future revenues in private and public markets
Tactics	Lobby for employer and individual mandates, and expansion of Medicaid
Rewards	Larger private and public markets
	Increased revenues ($170 billion), more than offsetting its pledged amount (40)

Organized Medicine

Pledge	No specific pledge
Agenda	Support private markets and restrain government intervention
	Prevent cuts in Medicare reimbursement
Tactics	Supports employer and individual mandates, insurance reforms, and expansion of Medicaid
	Opposes public option, rate-setting by independent commission, and targeted reimbursement cuts by specialty
Rewards	$245 billion "doc fix" restores Medicare reimbursement, at least for a time
	Increased revenues from expanded insured population

- Health care industries target both political parties in lobbying for their special interests. According to the Center for Public Integrity, by 2009 there were more than 4,500 lobbyists—eight for every member of Congress—attempting to influence the legislation. The lobbying industry had taken in $1.2 *billion* by the time the bill was passed.

- Meanwhile, of course, in this uncertain political climate, corporate stakeholders in our profitable market-based system continue to throw big money to legislators on a bipartisan basis. As Benjamin Page, professor of decision-making at Northwestern University, and Martin Gilens, professor of politics at Princeton University, tell us in their book, *Democracy in America? What Has Gone Wrong and What Can We Do About It*:

  > *We believe that both major parties tend to be corrupted—and pushed away from satisfying the needs and wishes of ordinary Americans—by their reliance on wealthy contributors. We see this reliance as one of the major reasons for today's feeble state of democratic responsiveness. It is one of the main reasons that so many Americans are so angry at politicians. No wonder most Americans tell pollsters that public officials "don't care much what people like me think."* [23]

III. Major Legislation During the Biden Administration (2021 - 2025)

The Biden administration clearly had the upper hand on what was apparently the single leading issue during the campaign. Inflation eased to a new three-year low of 2.5% in August 2024, giving the U. S. the most successful Covid-recovery economy in the world. Figure 3.1 shows the dramatic recovery course in the G7 since 2019 for seven developed countries.

Figure 3.1

Real GDP Recovery in the G7 Relative to Pre-Pandemic

Real GDP Recovery in the G7 Relative to Pre-Pandemic
Index, 2019 Q4 = 100

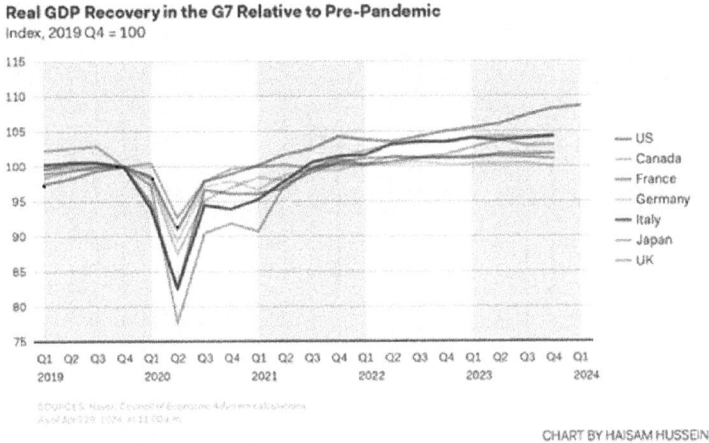

CHART BY HAISAM HUSSEIN

Four major bills were passed during the Biden administration:

1. *The American Rescue Plan:($1.2 trillion for maintaining and improving infrastructure, 2021);*
2. *The Chips and Science Act (2022); and*
3. *The Production of Cutting Edge Semiconductors Act) ($80 billion over next 10 years.); and*
4. *The Inflation Reduction Act (2022), with its subsidies and direct payments to support transition to a green economy, and with tax measures to cover its costs.*

As a result of these bills, the U. S. found inflation well controlled, growth in factory construction, increased sales on electric vehicles and wind and solar installations, and cost-effective clean energy with fossil fuels. Tax policy saw an increase of IRS enforcement policies, together with a new tax on stock buybacks to better rein in corporate profits.

Regulation was improved by the Federal Trade Commission's new head, Lisa Khan. Biden became the most pro-union President, walking the picket line during United Auto Workers' successful strike.

Dean Baker, senior economist and co-director of the Center for Economic and Policy Research and author of *Rigged: How Globalization and the Rules of the Modern Economy Were Structured to Make the Rich Richer*, congratulates Biden this way:

> Under Biden, the United States made a remarkable recovery from the pandemic recession. We have seen the longest run of below 4.0 percent unemployment in more than 70 years, even surpassing the long stretch during the 1960s boom. This period of low unemployment has led to rapid real wage growth at the lower end of the wage distribution, reversing much of the rise in wage inequality we have seen in the last four decades. It has been especially beneficial to the most disadvantaged groups in the labor market.[24]

In his final "farewell" address, President Biden warned America that our nation is succumbing to an oligarchy of the ultra-wealthy, at the same time as billionaires are calling for avoidance of fact-checking of social media, altogether a challenge to our democracy.

IV.   *What Next for Trump's Second Term?*

With a 180-day policy agenda, Project 2025's policy agenda includes plans for almost all federal agencies, with goals including ending diversity, equity and inclusion programs; imposing additional restrictions on abortion, opposing the FDA's approval of Mifepristone, and further restricting work requirements for food stamps.[25]

There is no question but that billionaire money played a large, if not decisive role in the outcome of the 2024 elections. Trump's choice of a billionaire hedge fund manager was his pick for Treasury Secretary, with the likely goal to maintain a rigged system that works for big corporations and the wealthy.[26] His agenda will include tax cuts, cutting spending, and enacting tariffs. Extension of his 2017 tax cuts will be a special challenge, since they expire in 2027, when revenue available for government spending will be reduced by about $2 to 4 trillion, a number that economists find alarming. [27]

The incoming Congress can be expected to pass legislation fitting their overall future goals. With tight House votes and a 53-47 Republican majority in the Senate, the GOP can be expected to combine as many priorities as possible into one bill in early 2025. This increasingly corrupt government will be one of crony capitalism, not competence, implementing government policy.

Conclusion

Having considered health care in both major political parties, together with the continuing growing role of billionaire money in determining the results of the 2024 elections, it is now time in Part III to address the many ways that conservative, corporate policies fight to retain their primary role in U. S. health care.

References:

1. FDR noted in his famous re-election speech in 1936.
2. Daniel Aubel, Legislation That Would Shape FDA And NIH Triggers Lobbying Frenzy November 25, *KFF Health News*, By Sydney Lupkin.
3. Health companies gave generously to President Trump's inauguration, *Kaiser Health News*, 21 April 2017.
4. Big Pharma's Government Revolving Door: 'Who Do They Really Work For?', *KFF Health News* Published Jan. 25 2018.
5. Thom Hartmann, Monopoly in Pharma: Big Private Profits from Publicly Granted Patents The Hidden History of Monopolies: How Big Business Destroyed the American Dream, *The Hartmann Report*, Mar 10, 2024.
6. Lilly Admits $1.4 Billion Zyprexa Mistake, Jan 15, 2009, Forbes Magazine.
7. PhRMA cut down to size By Ben Leonard, Grace Scullion and Ruth Reader, *Politico/AP*, 12/02/2022.
8. Jay Hancock, Drug Industry Spent Millions To Squelch Talk About High Drug Prices, December 19, 2017 *KFF Health News*.

9. How Much Could COVID-19 Vaccines Cost the U.S. After Commercialization? Jennifer Kates, Cynthia Cox, Josh Michaud, *KFF,* Mar 10, 2023.

10. Ethen Kim Lieser, Amazon Vendors Hiked Prices on 'Essential' Items During Pandemic, January 12, 2021, National Interest.org.

11. Mike Ludwig, New Report Shows Top Billionaires' Wealth Skyrocketing During Pandemic, *Truthout,* December 11, 2020.

12. Ibid.

13. New Study: Hospitals Hike Charges by Up to 18 Times Cost *National Nurses United,* November 16, 2020.

14. Harris Meyer, For-profit groups have vacuumed up over 70% of America's nursing homes, *KFF Health News,* March 12, 2024.

15. Cathy Schoen, Sara R. Collins, The Big Five Health Insurers' Membership And Revenue Trends: Implications For Public Policy, *Health Affairs,* December 2017.

16. Wendell Potter, Nation on the Take: How Big Money Corrupts Our Democracy and What We Can Do About It, *Kirkus Reviews,* March 1, 2016.

17. Medical Imaging Market Size, Share & Industry Analysis, *Fortune Business Insights,* March 31, 2025.

18. Geyman, J. P., *Do Not Resuscitate: Why the Health Insurance Industry is Dying, and How We Must Replace It,* 2008, *Common Courage Press,* 2008.

19. Consolidation in Hospital Sector Leading to Higher Health Care Costs, Study Finds Zarek Brot-Goldberg, Consolidation in Hospital Sector Leading to Higher Health Care Costs, Study Finds, *Harris School of Public Policy,* April 24, 2024.

20. Suzanne G Bollmeier, Scott Griggs,, The Role of Pharmacy Benefit Managers and Skyrocketing Cost of Medications, *National Library of Medicine,* Sept. 2024.

21. Medicare Advantage Will Be Overpaid by $1.2 Trillion, March 25, 2025, *Committee for a Responsible Federal Budget,* March 26, 2025.

22. Angie Drobnic Holan , https://www.npr.org/2009/08/21/112094043/public-option-divides-obama-insurance-industry, *Politifact - the Poynter Institute,* December 23, 2009.

23. Martin Gilens, professor at Princeton University, *Democracy in America? What Has Gone Wrong and What Can We Do About It, University of Chicago Press ,* December 22, 2009.

24. Dean Baker, The Biggest Success Story the Country Doesn't Know About, *New Republic.com,* July 29, 2024.

25. Maia Romanowska, Project 2025: Key Agenda Points and Expected Implementation Timeline, Maia's Substack, *einfodemic.substack.com*, Nov 06, 2024.
26. Meridith McGraw, Michael Stratford, Sam Sutton, Trump taps hedge fund manager Scott Bessent to lead Treasury, *Politico*, 11/22/2024.
27. Howard Gleckman, Sr. Contributor, No Matter The Accounting, Extending The 2017 Tax Cuts Will Cost Over $4 Trillion, *Forbes*, Feb 24, 2025.

PART III

WHY THE U. S. "SYSTEM" NEEDS REFORM

Big Business cares only about profit. With the rules that are currently in place. Big Business is encouraged to ruthlessly pursue profit at the expense of workers, communities, and the environment . . . Which raises a fundamental question asked from the days of Plato to Adam Smith to Bernie Sanders. Is the economy here to serve the majority of the people, or are the majority of people here to serve the economy and those few who own the largest parts of it? [1]

—Thom Hartmann, author of *The Hidden History of Monopolies: How Big Business Destroyed the American Dream*

Chapter 4

Increasing Privatization
of Health Care

*Making a profit from the most desperate is difficult,
even when the government pays. Those fellow citizens
who live on the margins, those in the lowest tenth in terms
of income, spend some 35% of their pre-tax income on
medical care. Those in the top 10% of income spend 3.5
percent . . . The obvious result is a group of people who
are sicker and poorer, so it's convenient for politicians
to do this in the name of the free market, efficiency, and
consumerism. It absolves them. But it also gives wealthy
corporations a license to radically transfer public funds
from the most desperate citizens to their CEOs and
shareholders.* [2]

–Cohen, D, Mikaelian, A. Authors of the 2021 book, *The Privatization
of Everything: How the Plunder of Public Goods Transformed
America* and *How We Can Fight Back.*

The above observation cuts to the heart of ongoing trends in
the increased privatization of U. S. health care. It is all based on a
long-standing myth, now a meme, that somehow the private sector
is more efficient and provides more value than the public sector.
This has been disproven in our country over many decades, but
privatization continues to be seriously detrimental to the public
interest.

This chapter has three goals: (1) to briefly bring some historical
perspective to this claim, which should have been abandoned
years ago in health care; (2) to describe the extent and results of
privatization of U. S. health care; and (3) to compare private vs. social
health insurance in terms of the extent to which they serve the public
interest.

I.   *Historical Perspective*

Medicare was the first public program to be privatized, aided especially after passage in Congress in 1982 of the Tax Equity and Fiscal Responsibility Act (TEFRA). That bill allowed Medicare to contract with HMOs and pay them 95 percent of what traditional Medicare would pay for fee-for-service (FFS) care in beneficiaries' county of residence. The claim at the time was that private was more efficient and less expensive, but this was just a "bait and switch" gambit. A gaming system was soon launched by which privatized Medicare would pay *much more* than for traditional Medicare.

By 1989, a report by Mathematica Policy Research, under contract to the Health Care Financing Administration (HCFA), found that Medicare was paying 15-33 percent more to private Medicare HMOs than for fee-for-service care in traditional Medicare.[2] Overpayments reached about $283 *billion* between 1985 and 2008.[3] Privatized Medicare received a big boost with the 1994 elections, when Republicans took control of both the House and Senate for the first time since 1954. Disregarding all experience with the grossly inflated costs of private Medicare programs, House Speaker Newt Gingrich, as part of the GOP's Contract with America, set out to hand over Medicare as a federal "entitlement program" to the private sector. In his famous words:

> *If we can solve Medicare, I think we will govern for a generation.* [4]

Here are three ways which show that the private sector in an unfettered health care marketplace fails to serve patients' best interests:

- According to a 2004 report, a nine-year tracking study of 12 major health care markets found these four barriers to efficiency of markets: (1) providers' market power; (2) absence of potentially efficient provider systems; (3) employers' inability to push the system toward efficiency and quality; and (4) insufficient competition among health plans.[5]
- Corporatization and consolidation have increased in recent years throughout the medical-industrial complex, including

among insurers, hospital systems, nursing homes, the drug industry, and dialysis centers. As their market shares grow, they have more latitude to set prices to what the traffic will bear.

- Responding to their shareholders, corporate stakeholders pursue the business "ethic" seeking maximal revenue well beyond the service tradition.

Today, more than one-half of Medicare's 55 million beneficiaries are now in private Medicare plans, as well as more than one-half of 66 million people enrolled in Medicaid. [6] The GOP still intends to further privatize and cut federal responsibility for Medicare and Medicaid as "entitlement programs," in an ongoing effort to reduce the growing federal deficit resulting from the GOP tax plan.

Joseph Stiglitz, Nobel Laureate in Economics and former chief economist at the World Bank, has noted the clash between markets and social justice in this way:

> *Markets do not lead to efficient outcomes, let alone outcomes that comport with social justice. As a result, there is often good reason for government intervention to improve the efficiency of the market. Just as the Great Depression should have made it evident that the market often does not work as well as its advocates claim, our recent Roaring Nineties should have made it self-evident that the pursuit of self-interest does not necessarily lead to overall economic efficiency.* [7]

II.   *Privatization Across U. S. Health Care*

Time after time, whatever part of our health care system we look at, we find that privatization brings higher costs, less efficiency, less service, more bureaucracy, profiteering and often corruption. Privatized companies and contractors keep coming back to the public till and taxpayers for more money as their inefficiencies mount, in every case disproving their claimed efficiencies. Figure 4.1 shows the extent of for-profit ownership of health care providers across our health care system as of 2016.

Figure 4.1

EXTENT OF FOR-PROFIT OWNERSHIP, 2016

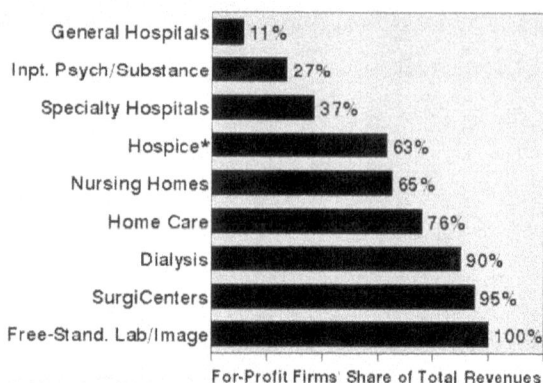

Category	For-Profit Firms' Share of Total Revenues
General Hospitals	11%
Inpt. Psych/Substance	27%
Specialty Hospitals	37%
Hospice*	63%
Nursing Homes	65%
Home Care	76%
Dialysis	90%
SurgiCenters	95%
Free-Stand. Lab/Image	100%

For-Profit Firms' Share of Total Revenues

Source: Commerce Dept. Service Annual Surveys and MedPac. Data are Q1, 2016 or most recent available. *Data are for share of establishments.

Let's take a look at how the private sector performs in five major areas of our health care system, with a view to how they serve their own self-interest vs. the public interest.

1. Medicare

The experience of privatized Medicare is a poster child for the abuses of corporate promises. The federal government has been very friendly to privatized Medicare in so many ways, including overpayments compared to traditional Medicare. The original idea that private Medicare plans would receive just 95 percent of fee for service fell by the wayside early on.

Overpayments to private Medicare plans reached $173.7 billion between 2008 and 2016, despite any attempts by the ACA to rein them in. [8] All of these overpayments can be traced to upcoding and other ways used by private insurers to inflate the severity of their enrollees' conditions. Compared to traditional Medicare, privatized Medicare plans have consistently been more expensive, less efficient, less reliable, more restrictive in choice of physician and hospital, and have administrative costs about five times higher. [9] Table 4.1 shows the major differences between privatized and public Medicare. Ongoing lobbying by corporate stakeholders has led Congress to turn a blind eye to these overpayments.

Table 4.1

COMPARATIVE FEATURES OF PRIVATIZED AND PUBLIC MEDICARE

PRIVATIZED MEDICARE	ORIGINAL MEDICARE
Experience-rated eligibility	Universal coverage
Managed competition	Social insurance as earned right
Defined contribution	Defined benefits
Segmented risk pool	Broad risk pool
Market pricing to risk	Administered prices
More volatile access & benefits	More reliable access & benefits
Increased cost sharing	Less cost sharing
Less accountability	Potential for more accountability
Less choice of provider & hospital	Full choice of provider & hospital
Less well distributed	Well distributed
Less efficiency, higher overhead	More efficiency, lower overhead

Source: Geyman, JP. *Shredding the Social Contract: The Privatization of Medicare.* Monroe, ME. *Common Courage Press*, 2006, p.206.

Here is how the private health insurers make all this loot through overpayments to Medicare, according to a very experienced physician who has followed this pattern over the years.

We found half a trillion dollars in overpayments by Medicare Advantage companies since 2007. They use two main strategies. Number one is making their patients look as sick as possible through aggressive coding. They have various tactics of diagnostic upcoding so that their customers look as sick as possible on paper. But then they use other strategies that lead to favorable selection—meaning they avoid the sicker Medicare enrollees, what people refer to as lemon dropping, and they try to find the most-healthy ones, which some people refer to as cherry picking. [10]

—Adam Gaffney, M.D., past President of
Physicians for a National Health Program

Ralph Nader added this further observation on virtually unseen practices by private health insurers:

> *Medicare Advantage would be a more accurate name for the programs, as insurance companies push to corporatize all of Medicare, yet keep the name for the purposes of marketing, deception, and confusion . . . Under Medicare Advantage, you are subject to all kinds of differing plans, maddening trapdoor fine print, and unclear meaning when insurers argue no "medical necessity" to deny care . . . All this anxiety, dread and fear, all these arbitrary denials of care—prompted by a pay-or-die commercial profit motive . . . The whole universal system costs half per capita of that in the U. S., where over eighty million people are uninsured or underinsured—still!* [11]

> —Ralph Nader, consumer advocate, founder of
> Public Citizen and the Center for Responsive Law,
> and author of *Out of Darkness: Essays on Corporate
> Power and Civic Resistance. 2012-2022, pp. 97, 99.*

Here is the bottom line of where Medicare stands today in terms of cost savings:

> *The seeds of Medicare's destruction are in the air. The program as it was set out in 1965 had kept millions of Americans out of medical poverty for over 50 years, but may well become something else–a privatized health care system for the oldest citizens whose medical care will depend on the profit goals of a handful of private insurers.*

> —Merrill Goozner, health columnist and
> former editor of *Modern Healthcare* [12]

Private Medicare plans game the system to avoid sicker, more costly enrollees, many of whom are dis-enrolled as their access is cut to preferred physicians, hospitals, and necessary drug treatment. From its beginning, both major political parties have assumed that

Medicare should be based in employer insurance and be mostly profit centered. It would be subsidized if needed by infusions of corporate funds in order to generate additional business, guarantee profits, and write off overhead while avoiding a public system. [13]

These are examples of progress toward their goals:

- Two thirds of Americans pay more in payroll taxes than they do in income taxes, mostly to Social Security and to support Medicare. [14]
- Despite the cooling of inflation, the cost of employer health insurance rose 7% for the second straight year in 2024, with the average family premium reaching $25,500. [15]
- Dr. Mehmet Oz, celebrity surgeon nominated by Trump to lead the Centers for Medicare and Medicaid Services has voiced support for expanding privatized Medicare Advantage, costing hospitals more. [16]
- Private equity investments ranged from acquiring hospitals, physician practices, nursing homes, mental health entities, home care services, hospices, and ambulance services. Costs routinely increase while quality and quantity of care decreases.[17]
- Private health insurers raise their prices by various hidden means, including substituting lesser trained providers for physicians and use of a pay-for-diagnosis system, including billing for services not provided. [18]
- In the first nine months of 2024, while its enrollment in commercial and Medicare Advantage plans increased, UnitedHealth Group made $24.5 billion in profits; that was due to the "unwinding" in the number of people enrolled in Medicaid that has been happening since the end of the COVID pandemic. [19]
- Physicians involved in United Health's system of turning diagnoses into profit centers could earn up to $30,000 a year while nurses tasked with "finding" new diagnoses were paid $250 per patient visit.[20]
- Starting February 1, 2025, Anthem Blue Cross Blue Shield will no longer cover anesthesia for the full length of certain surgical procedures if they exceed an arbitrary time set by the insurer. [21]

2.   *Medicaid*

Privatized Medicaid follows the same pattern as for privatized Medicare. One such example is Tennessee Medicaid plans, operated by Blue Cross BlueShield of Tennessee, UnitedHealthcare, and Anthem, with their inadequate physician networks, long waits for care, and denials of many treatments, even as these insurers take away more profits.[22] A 2016 report by auditors at DHHS's Office of Inspector General estimated that Florida paid about $26 million over five years for coverage of people who had already died, mostly as a result of outdated information on state databases and a lack of collaboration among different agencies. [23]

3.   *Veterans Administration*

After failing to fully repeal the ACA, deep-pocketed conservatives, driven by Koch money, have turned their sights on privatizing the VA, again falsely claiming that private would be more efficient. After 16 years of war, the already underfunded VA has been attacked for its long waiting times as the numbers of returning veterans with major medical and mental health problems increased their workloads. A battle has emerged between the majority of veterans and such long-standing organizations as Veterans of Foreign Wars and the American Legion and a new pro-privatization group, Concerned Veterans of America. [24]

The VA cares for almost 9 million veterans each year and has been more effective than private plans in improving quality of care, containing costs, and implementing electronic medical records. Table 4.2 shows how the quality of care in VA hospitals compares with non-VA hospitals, based on studies by RAND and the Agency for Healthcare Research and Quality (AHRQ). [25]

As well-funded conservative lobbyists pressed their case for privatizing the VA to congressional Republicans and the Trump administration, the Trump budget for the VA was 6 percent larger than last year's but one-third of the budget goes to private sector VA care, with only 1.3 percent to the VA itself. According to a 2017 wait

Table 4.2

Quality of Care in VA
Versus Non-VA Hospitals

Health Indicator	VA Score*	National Sample**
Overall	67%	51%
Chronic care	72%	59%
Lung disease	69%	59%
Heart disease	73%	70%
Depression	80%	62%
Diabetes	70%	47%
Hypertension	78%	65%
High cholesterol	64%	53%
Osteoarthritis	65%	57%
Preventive care	64%	44%
Acute care	53%	55%
Screening	68%	46%
Diagnosis	73%	61%
Treatment	56%	41%
Follow-up	73%	58%

* 596 VA patients ** 992 patients at non-VA hospitals
Data: RandCorp; Agency for Healthcare Research & Quality

Source: Arnst, C. The best medical care in the U.S. *Business Week*, July 17, 2006

time survey by Merritt Hawkins, wait times in the private sector, averaging about 24 days, are not much better than at a VA facility. Multiple polls have shown that a majority of veterans are satisfied with VA care and would rather see increased VA funding than money being funneled to the private sector. Will Fischer, a Marine Corps veteran who deployed to Iraq in 2004, brings us this insight:

> By making [private-sector care programs] mandatory, [VA officials] will be then pulling money out of other VA programs to fulfill the obligation of [private-sector programs] being mandatory—thus turning the VA into a slush fund for hospital executives and private care.[26]

4. *Mental Health Care*

We've had a long-term system problem in this country due to lack of parity of coverage between mental health and substance abuse problems and medical/surgical conditions. This situation led to passage by Congress of the Mental Health Parity and Addiction Act of 2008 (MHPAA). The intent of that law was to prevent group health plans from imposing less favorable limitations on those benefits than on medical/surgical benefits. Despite that legislation, this problem is ongoing. Milliman Inc., a national risk management and health care consulting company, in a study covering all 50 states and the District of Columbia, found that in 2015:

- Behavioral care was 4 to 6 times more likely to be covered by insurers out-of-network than for medical and surgical care.
- Insurers pay primary care providers 20 percent more for the same types of care as they pay mental health and addiction specialists.
- There is wide variation from one state to another; in New Jersey, 45 percent of office visits for behavioral health care were out-of-network.

As a result, because of the high proportion of out-of-network behavioral care, these patients are more likely to face high out-of-pocket costs, even with insurance, which for many are unaffordable. [27]

Partly because of insurers' reimbursement policies, there is a critical shortage of mental health and substance abuse professionals. Narrow behavioral health networks typically do not have enough therapists available.

To make matters worse, separately and without explanation, the Trump administration froze the National Registry of Evidence-based Programs and Practices (NREPP), which was launched in 1997 to help find effective interventions for preventing and treating mental illness and substance abuse disorders. [28]

There is another enormous problem that makes the care of mental illness and substance abuse disorders even more challenging—the under-recognized growth of privatized prisons. This trend started in the 1980s, and by 2008 private prisons were big business with about 18 corporations guarding 10,000 prisoners in 27 states. At that time, 16 percent of the nation's 2 million prisoners were mentally ill and would receive no treatment in prison. Wall Street investors have been happy with the profits that were possible by having the inmates work for as little as 17 cents per hour, or $20 per month for work up to 6 hours a day. The profit potential is further increased because so many people are being jailed for non-violent crimes, with long prison sentences for possession of microscopic quantities of illegal drugs, as well as passage of laws in some states that require minimum sentencing regardless of the circumstances. [29]

By 2018, for-profit private prisons were a $5 billion industry that controlled about 126,000 lives. They operated 65 percent of the country's detention beds. It was mostly opaque and almost entirely unaccountable.[30] Still another big problem is that private prisons prey on the poor and mentally ill, whereby poverty is criminalized by a mass incarceration system. The U. S. has more people in jail that anywhere else on the planet. Moreover, there is what turns out to be a loan shark operation to jail the poor for fines and bail. People are arrested on minor matters, held in jail on bail for $500, $1,000 or much more, must plead guilty when that is unaffordable, then squeezed by a payment plan. It is estimated that 10 million people nationally owe some $50 billion in court debt. [31]

5. EMS services

In the wake of the 2008-2009 recession, many cities and towns across the country struggled to afford ambulance services. Private equity stepped in as new private ambulance companies sprouted up with a mission to make as much money as possible from what should be a public service. A 2016 report from the *New York Times* exposed their bad practices that often endangered the lives of patients. As they cut costs, raised prices, and adopted aggressive billing practices, ambulances often had expired medications, problems with life-saving equipment, regular breakdowns, delayed response times, even with no ambulances available on some occasions. "E. R. shopping" was a common practice whereby ambulances raided E. R.s for supplies. [32]

III.   *The Ongoing Debate over Private vs. Social Health Insurance*

In its 1999 report, Medicare and the American Social Contract, a study panel of the National Academy of Social Insurance (NASI), noted these three key findings:

- Medicare was created as a response to a serious problem: The private market did not and could not work for a large population of the nation's elderly and disabled population.
- Medicare was originally designed as a social insurance
- Decisions about Medicare's future, including its ability to deal with health care utilization and costs, will not (and cannot) be made on purely economic or medical criteria.

Instead, seven criteria were recommended to be considered and weighed against each other as values and public concerns in the ongoing debate over Medicare's future: financial security, equity, efficiency, affordability over time, political accountability, political sustainability, and maximizing individual liberty. [33]

Traditional fee-for-service (FFS) Medicare has held fast to these criteria in providing universal coverage to seniors and disabled enrollees and has consistently performed much better than privatized Medicare across the board, as already mentioned, showing the devastating impact that privatization has had on health care costs since the early 1990s. [34]

With increasing privatization of public plans in a market-based health care economy, we see higher costs, less efficiency, more bureaucracy and less accountability compared to public programs. Continuing with Medicare as an example of this pattern, the 2017 Commonwealth Fund International Health Policy Survey of Older Adults in eleven countries found that "the U. S. elderly face a 'triple whammy' as they experience higher cost sharing, higher levels of economic vulnerability, and dramatically higher health care costs—with prescription drugs often two or three times as expensive in the United States as in the other countries studied. [35]

In their 2014 book, *Social Insurance: America's Neglected Heritage and Contested Future*, Theodore Marmor, Jerry Mashaw and John Pakutka draw this important conclusion about the need for more government involvement to counteract the adverse effects of "free market" policies in our health care:

> *In health care, the "invisible hand" [of the free market] fails to drive down costs, improve quality, or ensure distributional outcomes that are regarded as fair. We can tinker with the rules, regulations and payment schemes that govern medical care, but the forces that increase the demands for and supply of more care are relentless. Only powerful countervailing institutions can keep them under control. Only governments have the necessary authority, assuming they have the political will to use it.* [36]

A 2024 paper updated private health insurers' current ways of maximizing profits by selecting healthier patients (*cherry picking*) and avoiding less healthy patients (*lemon dropping*). [37]

Concluding comment

We are seeing ongoing corporate welfare in the medical-industrial complex, as in so many other parts of our economy. Because of the economic and political power of the private health insurance industry, we have yet to deal with the obvious advantages of universal coverage as can be provided under a system of not-for-profit social insurance, as we will discuss in Chapter 12. For now, let's look in the next chapter at how patient protections, as provided under the ACA, have been lost under the onslaught of Trump sabotage.

References:

1.   Hartmann, T. *The hated U. S. health care system is why government shouldn't be run like a business. Common Dreams,* December 9, 2024.

2.   Cohen, C, Mikaelian, A. *The Privatization of Everything: How the Plunder of Public Goods Transformed America and How We Can Fight Back.* New York. The New Press, 2021, pp. 172-173.

3.   General Accounting Office (GAO). Medicare: Reasonableness of Health Maintenance Organizations Not Assured. GAO/HRD-89-41. Washington D.C.: Government Printing Office, 1989.

3.   Trivedi, AN, Gribla, RC, Jiang, L et al. Duplicate federal payments to dual enrollees in Medicare Advantage plans and the Veterans Administration Health Care System. *JAMA* 308 (1): 67-72, 2012.

4.   Speech by Gingrich, 1978, PBS.org,

5.   Smith, DG. *Entitlement Politics: Medicare and Medicaid 1995-2001.* New York. *Aldine de Gruyter*, 2002: 71, citing Congressional Quarterly Almanac, 1995, p. 73.

6.   Jeannie Fuglesten Biniek, M. Freed, A. Damico, T.Neuman, Half of All Eligible Medicare Beneficiaries Are Now Enrolled in Private Medicare Advantage Plans, *KFF*, May 01, 2023

7.   Stiglitz, JE. Evaluating economic change. *Daedalus* 133/3, Summer, 2004.

8.   Osborn, R. Dody, MM, Moulds, D. et al. Older Americans were sicker and faced more financial barriers to health care than their counterparts in other countries. *Health Affairs*, November 15, 2017.

9.   Healthcare-NOW! Single-Payer Activist Guide to the Affordable Care Act. Philadelphia, PA, 2013, p. 22.

10. Gaffney, A. Interview by Ralph Nader. *Capitol Hill Citizen*, November/ December 2004: 38-39.

11. Nader, R., author of *Out of Darkness: Essays on CorporatePower and Civic Resistance.* 2012-2022, pp. 97, 99.

12. Lieberman, T. Goozner: Trump presidency could slash coverage as Harris pushes Medicare expansion. healthcareuncovered@substack.com, November 4, 2024.

13. O'Leary, W. Corporatization of American Health Care. *The Progressive Populist*, March 1, 2024., p. 16.

14. Krugman, P. How Trump could bankrupt Social Security, *New York Times,* October 25, 2024, p. A:25.

15. Evans, M, Ulick, J. Health premiums soar even as inflation is cooling. *Wall Street Journal*, October 15, 2024, p. A:2.

16. Wainer, D. Why Republican control is spooking hospitals. *Wall Street Journal*, November 29, 2024, p. B:10.

17. Webster, JR., Private equity and the ravaging of U.S. health care. *The Pharos*, Summer, 2024, pp. 31-34.

18. Weaver, C, Mathews, AW. Medicare watchdog faults home-visit pay. *Wall Street Journal*, October 24, 2024, P. A:1.

19. Potter, W. UnitedHealth group has made $24.5billion in profits this year (so on Wall Street. healthcareuncovered@substack.com.

20. Potter, W. WSJ: How UnitedHealth's diagnosis game rakes in billions from Medicare. <healthcareuncovered@substack.com, January 7, 2025.

21. Potter, W. Tick-Tock: Anthem Blue Cross Blue Shield's dangerous anesthesia policy <healthcareuncovered@substack.com>

22. Himmelstein, DU, Woolhandler, S. The post-launch problem: The Affordable Care Act's persistently high administrative costs. *Health Affairs Blog*, May 27, 2017.

23. Chang, D. Florida paid Medicaid insurers $26 million to cover dead people, report says. *Miami Herald*, December 13, 2016.

24. Kesling, B. Kochs to push to reshape VA services. *Wall Street Journal*, November 4-5, 2017.

25. Arnst, C. The best medical care in the U. S. *Business Week,* July 17, 2006.

26. Fischer, W. As quoted by Bernd, C. How the Koch-backed effort to privatize the Veterans Health Administration jeopardizes everyone's health care future. *Truthout*, July 2, 2017.

27. Sun, LH, Eiperin, J. Trump administration freezes database of addictionand mental health programs. *The Washington Post*, January 10, 2018.

28. Gold, J. If your insurer covers few therapists, is that really mental health parity? *Kaiser Health News*, November 30, 2017.

29. Pelaez, V. The prison industry in the United States: Big business or a new form of slavery? *Global Research*, January 25, 2018.

30. Eisen, LB. Private prisons lock up thousands of Americans with almost no oversight.

31. Karlin, M. Jailing the poor for fines and bail is a government-operated loan shark operation. *Truthout*, February 4, 2018.

32.   Ivory, D, Protess, B, Daniel, J. When you dial 911 and Wall Street answers, *New York Times*, June 25, 2016.

33.   National Academy of Social Insurance, *Medicare and the American Social Contract*, February 1999.

34.   Geyman, JP. *Shredding the Social Contract: The Privatization of Medicare*. Monroe, ME. *Common Courage Press*, 2006, p. 206.

35.   Osborn, R, Doty, MM, Moulds, D et al. Older Americans were sicker and faced more financial barriers to health care than their counterparts in other countries. *Health Affairs*, November 15, 2017.

36.   Marmor, TR, Mashaw, JL, Pakutka, J. *Social Insurance: America's Neglected Heritage and Contested Future*. Los Angeles, CA. *Sage Copress*, 2014, p. 128.

37.   Malinow, A. Ana Malinow on the case against Medicare Advantage. *Corporate Crime Reporter*, vol. 38, no. 40, October 14, 2024.

Chapter 5

Loss Of Patient Protections

Well, we are protecting pre-existing conditions. [The GOP health care bills in Congress in 2017] will be as good on preexisting conditions as Obamacare.

—President Donald Trump [1]

Another outright lie by Trump, talking about GOP bills in Congress in May 2017, which would have eliminated many of the patient protections of the Affordable Care Act. We saw in preceding chapters various ways by which the ACA has been sabotaged, together with shifting responsibility from the federal government to the states. These actions would remove protections assured by the ACA, such as its banning of health insurance rates based on preexisting conditions, coverage of essential health benefits without annual lifetime limits, and guaranteed renewability.

This chapter has three goals: (1) to describe the kinds of losses of patient protections as a result of Trump's executive orders and administrative policies of the Department of Health and Human Services (DHHS); (2) to discuss the impacts on patients of the loss of these protections; and (3) to update who has health insurance in the U. S. today.

I.   *Loss of Patient Protections*

As enacted in 2010, the ACA established that: "All marketplace plans must cover treatment for pre-existing medical conditions. No insurance plan can reject you, charge you more, or refuse to pay for essential health benefits for any condition you had before your coverage started. Once you're enrolled, the plan can't deny you coverage or raise your rates based only on your health."

These are some of the many ways that the Trump administration withered away most of these consumer protections of plans offered on the ACA's exchanges during his first term in office.

1. Pre-existing conditions

Under state waivers that will be passed out readily by DHHS under the Trump administration, insurers are free in many states to market plans that deny coverage for pre-existing conditions and/or to charge big hikes in premiums if coverage is offered. Common reasons for denial include such conditions as cancer, asthma, hepatitis, and depression. According to the Center for American Progress, premiums would increase by $4,340 for patients with asthma and by $28,660 a year for patients having breast cancer, thereby pricing many out of the marketplace. [2]

In 2015, the AARP estimated that about 40 percent of adults age 50 to 64 would have pre-existing conditions rendering their coverage difficult or impossible to get. Based in its study estimating how this problem would vary from one state to another before the ACA, Figure 5.1 gives us some idea as to how many people will be so affected across the country.

Figure 5.1

Percent of Adults 50-64 With a Declinable Preexisting Condition

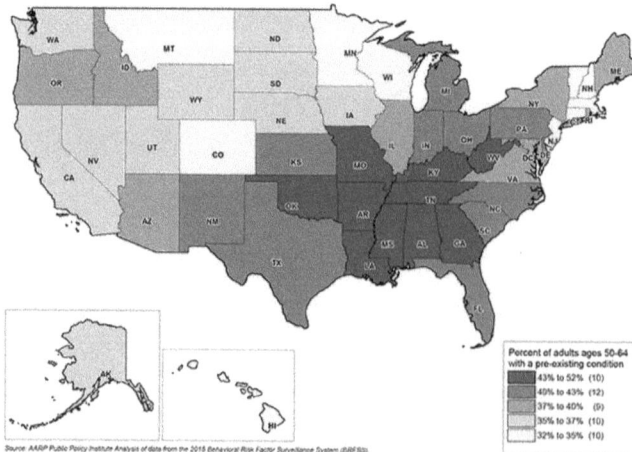

Figure 2: Percent of Adults Ages 50 to 64 with a Declinable Preexisting Condition under Pre-ACA Medical Underwriting Practices, 2015

Source: AARP Public Policy Institute Analysis of data from the 2015 Behavioral Risk Factor Surveillance System (BRFSS)

As Sabrina Corlette, research professor at Georgetown University's Health Policy Institute, observed:

> *The protection your insurance provides could depend a lot on where you live. In some states, over time, [patients with chronic illness] might find it increasingly difficult to find insurance companies that will offer plans that cover their needs.*[3]

The new landscape of Trumpcare would not pass the Jimmy Kimmel test, which evolved in the aftermath of his newborn son, Billy, born with a heart defect that required surgery and very large bills. On his late-night show, he made a passionate plea that "no parent should ever have to decide if they can afford to save their child's life." He invited Senator Bill Cassidy (R-LA), sponsor of the failed Graham-Cassidy bill in 2017, to his show, where they discussed the newly termed "Jimmy Kimmel test" - "No family should be denied medical care, emergency or otherwise, because they can't afford it." Though Sen. Cassidy seemed to agree with that notion on the show, his legislative effort would have failed to answer the affordability part, which in this instance could have reached lifetime cap territory.[4]

Dean Baker, senior economist at The Center for Economic and Policy Research, commenting on the Trump administration's attacks on the ACA:

> *To my view, the key part of Obamacare was creating a unified insurance market where anyone can get insurance regardless of their health and this is destroying that. So what this means is we'll be back to the world pre-Obamacare where, suppose you have a heart condition, suppose you are a cancer survivor, you either won't be able to get insurance at all or if you do have a company that's offering to sell you insurance, they're gonna want 50, 60, or 70,000 dollars a year . . . not many people could afford to pay that.*[5]

2. Increasing premiums

Average ACA exchange market premiums increased by 28 percent from 2014 to 2017.[6] Premiums will go much higher with deletion of the individual mandate and as insurers charge seniors five times as much as younger enrollees, compared to the 3:1 ratio of the ACA. Coverage will go down with promulgation of short-term, limited-coverage plans and association health plans, and other means by which the Trump administration had opened the door for insurers to expand new markets with "junk insurance." Short-term plans are expected to attract many healthy, young people, thus further segmenting risk pools and raising premiums for older and sicker people.

Insurers had already factored in the loss of CSR payments as they raised premiums for 2018. The consulting firm Avalere Health projected that premiums would go up by 69 percent in Iowa, 65 percent in Wyoming, and 64 percent in Utah. [6] A recent estimate by the Urban Institute projected that premiums for 2019 would increase by 18.2 percent in 41 states plus the District of Columbia. [7] Kevin Lucia, research professor and project director at Georgetown University's Health Policy Institute, predicted:

> *If consumers think Obamacare premiums are high today, wait until people flood into these short-term and association health plans. The Trump administration will bring rates down substantially for healthy people, but woe unto those who get a condition and have to go back into Obamacare.* [8]

3. Essential health benefits excluded

As we saw in Chapter 3, there are various ways that insurers can avoid coverage of any of the ACA's ten essential health benefits, especially through short-term limited-benefit plans and association health plans marketed to employers that cross state lines. Coverage would vary greatly from one state to another, and enrollees could expect to pay much higher out-of-pocket costs for health care. Enrollees would have to look carefully at the fine print of their plans to see what exclusions are built into their policies, such as whether chemotherapy is covered for patients with cancer. Insurers would also be able to exit insufficiently profitable markets without concern for their enrollees.

4.   New Medicaid restrictions

Some states are tightening their eligibility requirements, setting annual and/or lifetime caps (such as three to five years), and/or enforcing premiums with loss of coverage if not paid. Ten states have already applied for federal waivers to implement work requirements for their Medicaid recipients. Under Trumpcare, they will have these new ways to lose their coverage if they can't find work for various reasons—live in areas of persistent unemployment, got laid off during a recession, have seasonal jobs, or don't get enough work from their employer as they want. [9] Those who do not meet work requirements for Medicaid are unlikely to receive premium tax credits for plans offered on the ACA's exchanges, with many being unable to afford such coverage. [10] As Chad Bolt, senior policy manager at Indivisible, observed:

> Work requirements don't help the unemployed or underemployed to find work. [It] just punishes them when they're down—which is exactly what the Trump adminis-tration wants to do. [11]

In addition, implementing a work requirement policy for Medicaid adds a whole new layer of costly bureaucracy to the program.

II.   Impacts of Lost Patient Protections

Based on the above attacks on the ACA's protections, these are the inevitable consequences of the GOP's sabotage of the law without any replacement plan of their own.

1. Unaffordable premiums

The most popular ACA plans will see premium increases by an average of 34 percent in 2018. Molina Healthcare, one of the largest marketplace insurers, will increase its premiums by an average of 55 percent. [12]

2. Unaffordable care especially for older and sicker people

Even if insured, people will find their cost sharing increased for less coverage. As a result, they will pay more for actual care, if they can afford it at all. The proposed rule by DHHS for short-term, limited-duration plans even acknowledges that this coverage is "exempt from the ACA's individual market requirements because it is *not* individual health insurance coverage." Industry consultant Robert Laszewski predicts that we will have two different markets: a Wild West frontier called short-term medical . . . and a high-risk pool called Obamacare." [13]

3. Impacts on Medicare

The Trump budget released in February 2018 for fiscal year 2019 cut the budget of Medicare by $554 billion. Private Medicare Advantage plans covered about one-third of the 55 million people on Medicare. Sicker patients had to leave their plans as insurers cut access to preferred physicians, hospitals, and necessary drug treatment.

4. Impacts on Medicaid

Figure 5.2 shows the impacts of non-expansion of Medicaid in 2022. There are almost 25 million non-elderly adults enrolled in Medicaid. Although many gained coverage in the 32 states that expanded Medicaid under the ACA, most are still the usual population—children, people with disabilities, and non-elderly adults without Social Security. Nearly eight in ten of these Medicaid enrollees are in working families, and a majority are working themselves. Those who can't find work or are limited by disabilities will find themselves vulnerable to loss of coverage under Trumpcare's state waivers. Coming forward, almost one-half of states banning abortion would also oppose expansion of Medicaid, thereby further stressing the safety net.

Figure 5.2

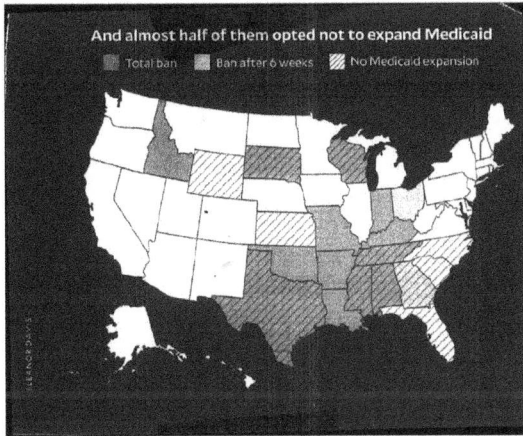

STATES BANNING ABORTION AND EXPANSION OF MEDICAID

Source: Kaiser Family Foundation, June 29, 2022 and July 7, 2022

5.   *More restricted networks*

This will happen as insurers cut providers to maximize profits, leaving many patients having to pay big increases in costs of out-of-network care.

6.   *Less choice*

Recall from the last chapter that there will soon be 454 counties with only one insurer with a growing number of counties with none.

7.   *Increased numbers of uninsured*

The CBO has projected that 13 million more people will be without health insurance by 2026, and this number is likely to be far higher as insurers in more states restrict their definition of essential health benefits. A March 2025 report from Medicare and Medicare Rights Center confirms that at least 12 million people will be harmed by planned cuts in 2025.

8.   *Increased numbers of underinsured*

Given the new freedom of insurers to market very skinny plans, we can anticipate tens of millions of people to be underinsured, all more a problem given the lack of cost and price constraints under Trumpcare.

9. Impacts on employer-sponsored insurance

Under association health plans, small businesses can join associations, based on certain kinds of professional, trade or interest groups in order to offer insurance across state lines with minimal standards for coverage. This will be another step toward increasing the numbers of underinsured.

10. Impacts on women's health care

These will be adverse as many insurers delete maternal health from their offerings. The GOP in many states has been cutting Planned Parenthood clinics and services, and that trend will likely continue. Already, the number of Planned Parenthood clinics across the country has been reduced from 860 to 600 in the last 13 years; prenatal services have been cut by more than two-thirds as the number of breast exams have been cut by almost one-half. [14]

11. Further fracturing of the nation's safety net

As responsibility for health care programs shifts to the states, we will see funding cuts to community health centers, hospitals, nursing homes and other safety net programs, including CHIP and SNAP (food stamps) because of lack of funds at the state level. Rural hospitals will be especially hard hit, with 83 closures already since 2010.

III.   Who Has Health Insurance Today in the U. S.?

We are indebted to the Commonwealth Funds's 2024 Biennial Health Insurance Survey to answer this question:

- 26 million Americans (8 percent of the population) were uninsured in 2023.
- Almost one in four Americans were *underinsured*, facing high out-of-pocket costs and deductibles that forced many to skip needed care or take on medical debt.
- 21 million people were insured under the ACA's market-based plans.
- 10 states have not adopted the ACA's Medicaid eligibility expansion.

- Many Americans with insurance are still burdened by medical debt, medical billing errors, or denial of coverage.
- Almost one-third of people with chronic conditions, such as heart failure or diabetes, skip medication doses or don't fill their prescriptions.[15]

Those numbers give us important background on how important the finding of full insurance coverage will be as we will see with national health insurance in the next chapter.

Concluding comment

Looking ahead to the second Trump administration, the policy agenda under Project 2025 calls for likely Medicare cuts, together with further work requirements, spending cuts, and time limits or lifetime caps on Medicaid benefits.

Many millions of Americans will be worse off than ever before as private health insurers enjoy another giveaway from the government. The unresolved question of how best to finance U.S. health care continues amidst the overlying statement of Benjamin Franklin when asked what kind of government we could foresee concerning the serious threat to our democracy:

A Republic, if you can keep it. [16]

References:

1. Trump, DJ. As quoted by Robert Dhondrup, *Liar-in-Chief: The Lies of President Trump.* May 1, 2017.
2. Pitt, WR. Graham-Cassidy is evil incarnate. *Truthout*, September 24, 2017.
3. Sabrina Corlette, Maanasa Kona, Lawsuit Threatens Affordable Care Act Preexisting Condition Protections But Impact Will Depend on Where You Live, Georgetown University, McCourt School of Public Policy. 2018
4. Yahr, E. Jimmy Kimmel gets heated about health-care bill, says Sen. Bill Cassidy 'lied right to my face.' *The Washington Post*, September 20, 2017.
5. Baker, D, as quoted by Wilpert, G. Will Trump's latest attack on Obamacare strike a death blow? *The Real News.com*, February 22, 2018.

6.	Research by Avalere, The high cost of healthcare: Patients see greater cost-shifting and reduced coverage in exchange markets 2014-2017. *Physicians for Fair Coverage.* , July 2018.

7.	Milbank, D. Trump just told the truth. He may wish he hadn't. *The Washington Post,* December 20, 2017.

8.	Lucia, K. As quoted by Appleby, J. Trump administration proposes rule to loosen curbs on short-term health plans. *Kaiser Health News*, February 20, 2018.

9.	Andrews, M. Refusing to work for Medicaid may not translate to subsidies for ACA plan. *Kaiser Health News*, February 27, 2018.

10.	Bolt, C. Trump launches 'truly savage' attack on Medicaid by pushing work requirement. *Common Dreams*, January 11, 2018.

11.	Mathews, AW. Molina to exit two exchanges. *Wall Street Journal*, August 3, 2017.

12.	Azar, A. Trump administration works to give relief to Americans facing high premiums, fewer choices. U. S. Department of Health & Human Services, February 20, 2018.

13.	Laszewski, R. As quoted by Appleby, J. Trump administration proposed rule to loosen curbs on short-term health plans. *Kaiser Health News*, February 20, 2018.

14.	Firozi, PW. Planned Parenthood goes on the offensive. *The Washington Post*, February 14, 2018.

15.	Collins, SR, Gupta, A. The State of Health Insurance Coverage in the U. S.: *Commonwealth Fund*, November 2024.

16.	Founding Father Benjamin Franklin, 1787, at Constitutional Convention. Progressive Democrats of America.

Useful Resources:

1.	Hancock, J, Bluth, R. Promises made to protect preexisting conditions prove hollow. *Kaiser Health News*, June 22, 2017.

2.	Hiltzik, M. The stupidity of TrumpCare: Government will spend $33 billion more to cover 8.9 million fewer Americans, as premiums soar. *Los Angeles Times*, February 26, 2018.

3.	Rosenbaum, S, Wachino, V, Gunsalus, R et al. State 1115 proposals to reduce Medicaid eligibility: Assessing their scope and projected impact. *The Commonwealth Fund*, January 11, 2018.

4.	Potter, W., While United Health Reports GIllions in Profits, Americans face 200% increases in out-of-pocket costs over last decade. *Wendell Potter NOW,* January1, 2022.

5.	Carter, J., New revenues show House budget would slash Medicaid, despite support of program. *Medicare Rights Center*, March 6, 2025.

Chapter 6

Declining Access To Affordable Health Care

Health care is a social good, not a commodity, just like primary education, fire and police protection, and clean water. A market-based system is not only wasteful, it's immoral.

—Dr. Marcia Angell, former editor-in chief of the *New England Journal of Medicine* [1]

This chapter will describe the various ways by which Trumpcare is certain to fail to meet the needs of Americans for affordable, quality health care.

Republicans are correct that the ACA left many needs unfulfilled, despite its success in bringing significant improvement to many millions of Americans. But everything Republicans have done to unravel the ACA, mostly by administrative means of the Trump administration, has made the situation far worse with no hope for improvement in sight. Trump's promises are hollow, disingenuous, and blatantly dishonest in touting what Trumpcare can do for us.

This chapter has three goals: (1) to describe eight different ways in which Trumpcare puts access to affordable care out of reach for much of the middle class as well as lower-income people; (2) to summarize health care costs today; and (3) to briefly discuss how increasing inequality in American society further contributes to inadequate access to health care.

I.   *The Many Barriers to Affordable Health Care*

1. The uninsured

We are indebted to the ongoing work of the Commonwealth Fund for what is happening in today's health care in this country. Its 2024 Biennial Health Insurance Survey found that:

- 26 million Americans (8% of the population) were uninsured in 2023.
- 56% of U. S. working-age adults were insured all year with adequate coverage to ensure affordable access to care.
- Among adults who were insured all year but still underinsured, 66% had coverage through their employer, 16% were in Medicaid or Medicare, and 14% had a plan purchased in the marketplaces or the individual market.
- 57% of the underinsured avoided getting needed health care because of the cost.
- Two of five adults who delayed or skipped care say it led to worsening of their health problems. [2]

Here is one example of what these abstract numbers mean to real people, which would be understandable in a third world country but not in this country with all its abundance.

Sarai was 25 years old when she died of Wilson's disease, an inherited disorder that leads to liver failure. She could have been cured by having a liver transplant, but was uninsured and was denied at two prominent liver transplant hospitals in Chicago for lack of coverage. Her physician signed her death certificate as liver failure but noted that the real cause of death was inequality. [3]

The early retired, not yet eligible for Medicare, give us other examples of people without access to affordable care despite their higher income levels. They are healthy people who have always bought their own health insurance but are now confronted with big premium hikes and high cost-sharing without being able to qualify for tax credits under the ACA. [4]

> *Teri Goodrich, 59, and her husband, John Kistle, 57, of Raleigh, North Carolina bought health insurance through their state's exchange for three years, but cancelled their insurance when premiums reached $19,200 a year with deductibles of $7,500 each. They later purchased short-term coverage, non-compliant with the ACA, for limited catastrophic coverage. As they said, 'We're getting slammed. We didn't budget for this'* [5]

2. The underinsured

Even with the ACA, we already have an epidemic of underinsurance in this country with 31 million people finding themselves without coverage when they need it despite paying more every year for premiums, deductibles, copayments, coinsurance, and out-of-pocket costs. The Commonwealth Fund defines underinsurance as households spending 10 percent or more of their annual income on medical care (not including premiums). It has also found that more than two of five underinsured Americans cannot afford to seek needed health care.[6] Under the Trump administration's stealth sabotage of the ACA, the word "insurance" continues to be meaningless. Even if "insured" with a short-term or bronze plan, people will be worse off than ever, especially because health care costs will continue to soar unabated in a deregulated marketplace.

3. Can't afford health insurance

As we saw in the last chapter, premiums in 2019 were expected to go up by more than 60 percent in some states, with an average of an 18 percent increase across the country.

Figure 6.1 shows what the U.S. spent in health care and Medicaid from 1966-2015. But these premiums bought less and less coverage. Insurers will entice some people to buy junk policies by offering them at low premiums, but the protection they will provide will be minimal and not qualify as actual insurance.

Figure 6.1

Total U.S. Health Spending And Medicaid Spending, 1966-2015

Total U.S. Health Spending (Billions)

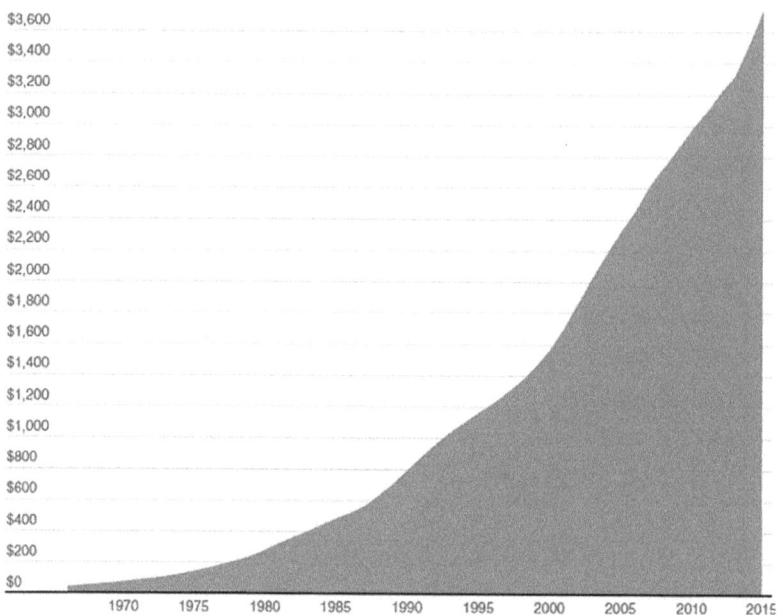

Source: Centers for Medicare & Medicaid Services

Here is what two middle class families in Charlottesville, Virginia, found when they went shopping for coverage on HealthCare.gov in November 2017:

> *Sara Stovall, 40, does customer-support work for a small software company. After researching her options on HealthCare.gov, she found that premiums for her family of four would triple to $3,000 a month with a deductible of $12,000, way beyond her ability to pay. She had been a believer in the ACA, but said 'It's not working as it was supposed to. It's being sabotaged, and I feel like a pawn.'*

> Ian Dixon, 38, works as a developer of mobile apps. Even though he does not need an assistant, he has considered hiring an employee just so he could buy health insurance as a small business at a cost less than what he and his family would pay on their own. He found two options on HealthCare.gov: (1) a plan with premiums of about $37,000 a year, with a deductible of $9,200 a year; or (2) a plan with annual premiums of $30,000 with a higher deductible of $14,400 a year. [7]

4. Cost sharing too high

Cost sharing with enrollees in health insurance plans has been a long-held mantra among conservatives, believing that patients with "more skin in the game" will be more conscious of costs and make more prudent decisions about their own health care. This premise has been completely disproven by experience over decades as ineffective in containing health care costs. But the disproven belief continues in TrumpCare with deductibles, copayments and other forms of cost sharing still widespread through the insurance market, even in privatized public programs.

> Paul Melquist and his wife in St. Paul, Minnesota are both 59. Paul worked in the defense industry and retired at the end of 2016. He delayed his retirement due to rising costs of health insurance, but was shocked to find they are even worse than he'd imagined. They pay $15,000 a year in premiums for a bronze plan with the first $6,550 for each of them for health care expenses out-of-pocket. So they end up having to pay out some $30,000 a year before anything gets covered. As Paul says, 'It's not that my life is falling apart, but the Affordable Care Act has ruined a lot of things I'd like to have done, [including being better able to help pay for his grandchildren's college expenses].' [8]

The cruel downside of increasing cost sharing is illustrated by the recent, possibly preventable death, of an elementary school teacher in Weatherford, Texas.

Heather Holland, 38-year old married mother of two, fell ill with what was thought to be the flu, but did not pick up a flu medication because she felt the $116 copay was too high. Her symptoms worsened several days later, she ended up in the ICU, was put on dialysis, and died about two days later. [9]

Although we can never know whether the medication could have prevented her death in this instance, we do know that many patients delay or forgo needed care because of high cost-sharing and incur worse outcomes.

5. Seniors having trouble affording care

Although Medicare has been a solid rock for more than 50 years in what has become a volatile and unstable health insurance market in this country, seniors still have trouble affording their health care costs. Seniors' out-of-pocket spending consumed 41 percent of Medicare beneficiaries' per capita Social Security income, on average, in 2013. [10] One in four seniors have problems getting care because of costs. [11]

The GOP and Trump's first administration made these problems markedly worse, again mostly by administrative policies led by CMS. Seema Verma, head of CMS, had long been a proponent of privatizing Medicare, as had House Speaker Paul Ryan. They wanted to convert traditional Medicare into a voucher program, eliminating the long-standing social contract with the elderly for universal access to care. The administration has already changed its premium policy to allow insurers to charge seniors five times as much as younger people, not the 3:1 ratio set by the ACA. Under a voucher system, private insurers could tailor their benefits to attract younger and healthier seniors, leaving sicker seniors in a higher risk pool with much higher costs, thereby threatening a death spiral for traditional Medicare. [12]

6. Restrictive Medicaid changes

With repeal and replacement of the ACA sidelined, at least for now, more states are requesting waivers from DHHS to implement their own policies, which may include work requirements, imposing premiums, lockout from coverage for non-payment or not updating changes in income quickly enough, and lifetime limits for Medicaid.

As we saw in the last chapter, premiums in 2019 were expected to go up by more than 60 percent in some states, with an average of an 18 percent increase across the country.

The work requirement is particularly regressive in that most Medicaid beneficiaries are already working; many who don't are caregivers, in school, unable to work because of illness or disability, or can't find a job in their area.

All of these changes would have more adverse outcomes if Trump's proposed budget cut in 2019 of almost half a trillion dollars over the next ten years took effect for the three pillars of the social safety net: Medicaid, federal housing assistance, and SNAP, the food stamp program. According to the Center on Budget and Policy Priorities, there are an estimated 5.7 million Americans that would be put at risk of hunger or homelessness if these budget cuts go forward. Here is what that would mean for one family struggling to stay afloat.

> *Daisy Franklin, a 60-year old grandmother in Norwalk, Connecticut, with her household of four, relies on Medicaid, a federal housing voucher, and more than $300 a month in food stamps. She had worked for decades assembling electronic components for local manufacturers, but had to stop after developing fibromyalgia. She now is on disability, collecting $1,250 a month, and cares for her adult daughter's two young children while she supplements the household income with a $10 an hour part-time job. Even with the disability check, food stamps, and a housing voucher that covers two-thirds of their $1,450 a month rent, their money is close to running out at the end of the month. As Daisy says: 'There's a lot of families in our same boat. People are afraid. They don't know what's going to happen to them.'* [13]

7. Annual and lifetime limits

The costs of today's high-tech medicine has put many of us at risk for enormous costs that can lead to our bankruptcy for a single major illness or accident. Many insurers are setting annual and lifetime limits for coverage. It may at first seem that a $1 million lifetime limit would be enough, but it will not turn out that way for many patients and families in today's market of runaway costs.

8. Trouble paying medical bills

In 2016, one-third of non-elderly Americans reported problems paying their medical bills, which are now the most common reason for receiving a debt collection phone call. There is a large and growing debt collection industry that often results in the arrest and jailing of many patients, with little protection from state courts and local prosecutors.[14]

According to a recent report from the ACLU, *A Pound of Flesh: The Criminalization of Private Debt*, one in five Americans has unpaid medical bills that have gone to collection. There are large and growng debt collection agencies operating in the country, collecting billions of dollars each year. The ACLU has found instances in which threatening letters have been sent for bounced checks as low as $2.00. The criminalization of private debt happens when judges issue arrest warrants for people who failed to appear in court, often when they were unaware of receiving such notice. Many people miss their court dates because of work, childcare responsibilities, physical disability, illness, lack of transportation, or because they didn't receive notice of their court date. Although Congress abolished debtors' prisons in 1833, look at what is still going on:

> Denise Zencka, mother of three, was arrested in Indiana in 2013 for non-payment of medical bills incurred from cancer treatment. She lived with her parents in Florida for several months during her recovery, during which—unbeknownst to her—she had been ordered to appear in small-claims court in Indiana. Three arrest warrants were issued when she failed to appear. She had already filed for

bankruptcy when she was arrested and jailed—in a men's mental health unit because she was physically unable to climb the stairs to the women's section.

A Georgia woman was arrested while caring for her terminally ill mother. She had a 6-year-old rental debt that her landlord claimed she owed after evicting her from her trailer home. She was jailed overnight. Her mother died two days later. [15]

III. *Total Health Care Spending Today*

Current health care spending was released by the Centers for Medicare and Medicaid Services that tells us a lot about how it all works. These are some of the major highlights today, still subject to the processes described above: [16]

National health care spending increased 7.5% year over year in 2023 to $4.867 trillion ($14,570 per person):

- Total spending on health care goods and services accounted for 17.6% of our gross national product;

- Spending on hospital care grew at the fastest pace since 1990;

- Just over one half of the population (175.6 million) had employer-sponsored insurance;

- 65 million Americans were on Medicare and almost 92 million were on Medicaid;

- The average worker spent almost 20% more on health insurance in 2023 compared to five years earlier (almost double that of ten years ago;

- Factors increasing health care costs included higher costs for hospitals and physicians' offices, consolidation among hospitals, and facility fees for outpatient facilities;

- Nine states would be at risk for losing Medicaid coverage if federal funding of their Medicaid expansions were to end. [17]

As we recall from Chapter 5, private insurers have no trouble in their quests for higher profits despite their complicated roles. Privatized Medicare and Medicaid have long been profitable for them. Private health insurers point to these kinds of factors to explain where they start in terms of profit negotiations:

- Upcoding by providers, especially hospitals, including by *their own negotiated agreements with middle-men;*
- increased spending on specialty drugs;
- and insufficient government funding of their rising costs. [18]

With the incoming second term of the Trump administration, we have to remind ourselves that the goals for health policy under Project 2025 will codify and make worse many of the so-called "value-based" payment mechanisms. As outlined in Dr. Jim Kahn's excellent description, it is designed to:

> *Increase the role of for-profit insurers, place a greater burden on individuals to pay for care, and cut public funding for health care for the poor, seniors, and the disabled. This will mean more medical debt and bankruptcies, less access to care, and worse health. The plan also targets abortion access, even where legal.* [19]

Project 2025 will also take on these kinds of approaches:

1. End the Affordable Care Act's regulation of private health insurance;
2. Increase the use of health savings accounts (HSAs);
3. Reduce health insurance coverage for the poor by restricting both eligibility and benefits;
4. "Reform" Medicaid funding by using "balanced" match rates, block grants and through fixed funding.
5. Cover only the sickest and poorest.
6. Use Medicaid to restrict access to abortion.

7. Use Medicaid money to support HSAs instead of public insurance.
8. End drug price negotiations; lower the Medicare role for catastrophic drug costs.

III. Declining Access due to Inequality

Inequality within our population has been increasing at an ever-faster rate in recent years. According to a report from Heather Boushey, Executive Director of the Washington Center for Equitable Growth, almost two-thirds of tax cuts from the GOP's tax bill of 2017 went to the top 20 percent. The top 1 percent of earners in 1980 took in 27 times more income than the bottom 50 percent. Since then that multiple has tripled to at least 80. [20]

The growing proportion of our society with limited incomes is increasingly vulnerable to worse health outcomes due to declining access to care. As Dr. David Ansell, former chief of general medicine at Cook County Hospital in Chicago for 17 years and author of *The Death Gap: How Inequality Kills*, says of his 40 years in medicine:

> *Our current multi-payer for-profit health insurance system perpetuates premature death by putting many people at an extreme disadvantage when it comes to affording care. Those who have better health insurance policies can access better care. However, even patients with insurance cards face skyrocketing copays, deductibles and pharmaceutical prices that keep them from seeking care. Last year, 27 percent of Americans said they had postponed or avoided getting care they needed because of the cost; 23 percent said they had skipped a recommended test or treatment due to cost; and 21 percent said they had chosen not to fill prescriptions for medication because they couldn't afford it. . . . Death rates tell the same story. Since 1980, there have been dramatic gains in life expectancy for the top 20 percent of U. S. earners. At the same time, the poorest 20 percent have seen their life expectancy plummet.* [21]

Concluding comment:

As Dr. Angell observed in her opening quote, this situation is immoral. Michael Corcoran of *Truthout* adds this important further conclusion:

> *Until the United States adopts a model of social insurance that provides health care to all, regardless of income, the poor will continue to be treated like collateral damage in the war against equality and justice.* [22]

This chapter has shown us how Trumpcare is an unmitigated disaster for much of our population, all under the lie that we will see better care for all of us! As we will see in later chapters, having "health insurance" has become more and more volatile and inadequate.

References:

1. Angell, M. The benefits of Bernie Sanders's 'Medicare for All' plan, *Boston Globe*, September 21, 2017.

2. Collins, SR, Gupta, A. The State of Health Insurance in the U. S.Commonwealth Fund 2024 Biennial Health Insurance Survey. November 21, 2024.

3. Collins, SR, et al. How the Affordable Care Act has improved Americans ability to buy health insurance on their own. Commonwealth Fund, February 1, 2017.

4. Ansell, D. I watched my patients die of poverty for 40 years. It's time for single payer. *The Washington Post*, September 13, 2017.

5. Rovner, J. Overlooked by ACA: Many people paying full price for insurance 'getting slammed.' *Kaiser Health News*, October 9, 2017.

6. Ibid # 4.

7. Issue Brief. The problem of underinsurance and how rising deductibles will make it worse. Findings from the Commonwealth Fund Biennial Health Insurance Survey, 2014. *The Commonwealth Fund*, May 20, 2015.

8. Pear, R. Middle-class families confront soaring health insurance costs. *New York Times*, November 16, 2017.

9. Ibid # 4.

10. Cubanski, J, Neuman, T, Smith, KE. Medicare beneficiaries' out-of-pocket health care spending as a share of income now and projections for the future. *Kaiser Family Foundation*, January 2018.

11. Osborn. R, Doty, MM, Moulds, D et al. Older Americans were sicker and faced more nancial barriers to health care than counterparts in other countries. *Health Affairs*, November 15, 2017.

12. Richtman, M. GOP's proposed Medicare voucher program would lead to demise of the system. *The Hill*, March 5, 2018.

13. Dewey, C, Jan, T. 'We would literally not survive': How Trump's plans for the social safety net would affect America's poorest. *The Washington Post*, February 14, 2018.

14. Turner, J. *A Pound of Flesh: The Criminalization of Private Debt. American Civil Rights Union*, 2018.

15. Germanos, A. New report details how Americans who have debt held by collection agencies can get thrown in jail. *Common Dreams*, February 21, 2018.

16. Torry, H. Nation's healthcare tab is surging amid rising wages, hospital fees, *Wall Street Journal*, December 20, 2024, p. A:3.

17. Gallewitz, P. Nine states poised to end coverage for millions if Trump cuts Medicaid funding. *The Progressive Populist*, Jan. 1-15, 2025, p.8.

18. Boushey, H. The tax bill should've been called the Inequality Exacerbation Act of 2017. *The Hill*, December 22, 2017.

19. Kahn, J. Project 2025 health policy critique redux. *Health Justice Monitor*, August 15, 2024.

20. Geyman, JP. *Shredding the Social Contract: The Privatization of Medicare.* Monroe, ME. *Common Courage Press*, 2006, p. 206.

21. Osborn, R, Doty, MM. et al. Older Americans were sicker and faced more financial barriers to health care than their counterparts in other countries. *Health Affairs*, November 15, 2017.

22. Corcoran, M. A legal battle is mounting against the GOP's attack on Medicaid. *Truthout*, February 6, 2018.

Chapter 7

Abortion and
Reproductive Rights

*The Supreme Court continues to do all the things that
Republicans cannot persuade voters to do, and further . . .
Either we expand the Supreme Court and break the conservative majority, or we accept that women and pregnant
people are second-class citizens who will lack equal access to
healthcare for a generation. That is the world that we live in,
and the people who deny it are selling you a fantasy.*[1]

—Elie Mystal, attorney and justice
correspondent for *The Nation*

One controversial ruling by the conservative U.S. Supreme
Court became a leading issue in the 2024 election campaigns.
The 2022 ruling struck-down a 1973 Roe v. Wade ruling that had
established a constitutional right to abortion in this country.

This chapter takes on three objectives: (1) to briefly consider
the initial implications of this SCOTUS ruling; (2) to discuss other
state-based bills being passed for other reproductive rights, including
medication abortion and in vitro fertilization; and (3) to consider
their fallout in national and state election campaigns.

I.   *Action by the U. S. Supreme Court*

Ballot measures on abortion rights have succeeded beyond
all expected projections since SCOTUS overturned Roe v. Wade
three years ago. Ten states asked voters whether or not to establish a
right to abortion in their constitutions, with abortion rights always
running in a lead position.

Today's legal questions over whether to proceed with urgently needed abortion legislation raise questions about who should make these decisions—women and their physicians or the judiciary in some states. When brought to legal recourse, seven states by 2024 had already affirmed abortion rights for women—California, Kansas, Kentucky, Michigan, Montana, Ohio and Vermont.[2] The Dobbs decision and the abortion bans to follow in some states led to *an increase* in the number of abortions being performed in this country, especially through telehealth.

Critics of SCOTUS have called its abortion ruling in 2022 an instance of "judicial activism" by depriving women of basic rights as assured by the history, text and structure of the U. S. Constitution. That fight brought up the legality of sending abortion medications by mail to patients based on an 1873 law, the Comstock Act, that labelled such materials as "obscene and immoral." [4]

The basic issue had become who could answer women's questions as to how to proceed with issues related to their individual decisions to proceed with a pregnancy—their own private discussions with their physicians and families or some government bureaucrat, varying by state? According to the Pew Research Center, 60 percent of Americans believe that abortion should be legal in all or most cases. [5]

II.   *Other Reproductive Rights*

As the 2024 election campaigns drew to a close, other related bills in state courts took center stage as well, especially in swing states. Bills on abortion led to related bills at the state level on other aspects of reproductive rights. The issue had become competing bills in states vs. a possible future national ban on abortion. Presidential candidate Trump tried to deny support for any specific bill as he distanced himself from the Project 2025 GOP guidebook.

In Vitro

The life of the embryo, as extended to in vitro services, had joined the national debate over abortion. In 2021, some 97,000 infants were born this way in the U. S. According to the Center for Reproductive Rights. So-called personhood bills have been passed by at least 13 states based on the premise that life begins at conception. Those bills would render illegal the practice of destroying embryos during the IVF process.[6] As an example, a State Court ruling in Alabama found that frozen embryos should be considered children.[7]

The fight over abortion rights also raised the legality of sending embryos by mail to patients based on an 1873 law, the Comstock Act, that labelled such materials as obscene and immoral. That law, still on the books, made it a federal crime to "send or receive materials designed, adapted or intended for obscene or abortion causing purposes." Fully aware that further legislative changes may well lead to another ruling by the U. S. Supreme Court, Congressional Republicans for these restrictive policies were aware that they still had the Comstock Act in their back pocket to defend these policies, including fetal personhood as part of the U. S. Constitution. [8]

Medication abortion

Contraception became another variant of reproductive rights seeing action in the states. Medication abortion is usually safe and effective, with just 3% to 5% of women needing another dose of mifepristone or a surgical D. and C.

One in five women of reproductive age living in states where abortion is banned has either struggled to get access to an abortion or know someone who has.[8] Mifepristone is part of a safe two-drug regimen to end pregnancies up to 10 weeks of gestation. A recent study by the Guttmacher Institute has shown a national *increase* in the numbers of abortions in the U. S. after the Dobbs decision, enabling 7,700 abortions a month in states with six-week bans or total abortion bans.[9]

Figure 7.1 shows how abortion had become the number 1 leading issue among suburban women in the U. S. for the 2024 elections, far ahead of inflation and immigration.

Figure 7.1

STATES WHERE ABORTION IS LEGAL, BANNED OR UNDER THREAT

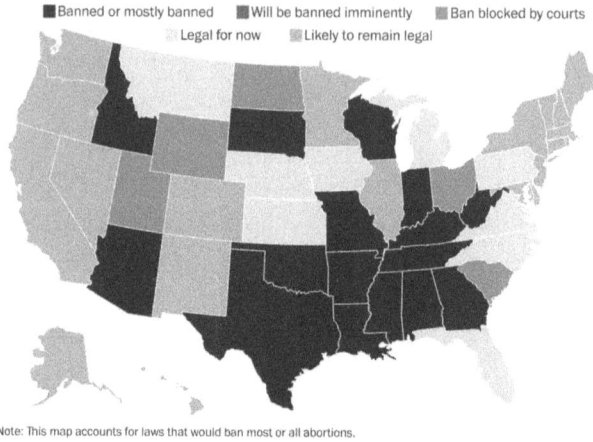

Note: This map accounts for laws that would ban most or all abortions.

Source: *The Washington Post*, June 24, 2022

As the number of abortion clinics declined and as vigorous protests were being held across the country, President Biden stepped up enforcement of the Freedom of Access to Clinic Entrances Act. Meanwhile, as RFK Jr. has become head of the Department of Health and Human Services, it appears that he would leave it to the states to decide future decisions about abortion rights. [10]

The debate over abortion raises confusion about its goal concerning pro-life vs pro-birth. Dr. Hal Lawrence, as CEO of the American College of Obstetricians and Gynecologists, notes:

> *The strange thing about this is that people who want to decrease the number of abortions are taking away access to the very services that help prevent them.*[11]

Sister Joan D. Chittister, O.S.B., social worker and author of the 2015 book, *Between the Dark and the Daylight*, adds:

> *I do not believe that just because you're opposed to abortion, that makes you pro-life. I think in many cases, your morality is deeply lacking if all you want is a child born but not fed, not a child educated, not a child housed. And why would you think that I don't? Because you don't want any tax money to go there. That's not pro-life. That's pro-birth. We need a much broader conversation on what the morality of pro-life is.*[12]

III. Election Results in National and State Elections

The November 2024 elections concluded with Donald Trump winning a second presidential term by the barest of margins. The leading issues were the economy and jobs. Republicans gained control of the Senate and also barely control of the House of Representatives.

According to follow-up reports from the Kaiser Family Foundation, these were the highlights of voter results on abortion policy and reproductive rights:

- These ranked high among voters, but not the leading issue among the electorate, among whom the economy took first place.

- 22 states with bans to abortion in all or most cases.

- Voters won key electoral victories in four states where voters chose to expand or protect abortion access.

- Voters in seven states voted to expand abortion access through abortion-related ballot measures, while abortion access failed in three states (Florida, South Dakota and Nebraska). [13]

- Three in ten women said the abortion policy was the "single most important" factor in their vote.[14]

Some filings by social media sites were found to suppress or confuse their postings on abortion services.[14] Apple is facing regulatory concerns from the European Commission, the European Union's antitrust authority, as to whether or not its postings meet the standards of its new Digital Markets Act.[15]

Unfortunately, legal uncertainties have raised the difficulties of pregnant women urgently needing an abortion to have to seek care in other states. It may be against the law for them to receive evaluation and treatment in their home state, even as they are bleeding out under emergency circumstances. In some states, such as in Texas, state laws hold their physicians at risk for losing their license if they provide care.[16]

This ongoing legal impasse has not only led to physicians in obstetrics and gynecology leaving their states, but also a new crisis in the numbers of medical students seeking future practice in these specialties. The U. S. thereby joins a recent report that has found that 45% of 73 million abortions worldwide are unsafe.[17]

Conclusion

Once again, as we have seen in previous chapters, the U. S. fails to lead in quality of care in abortion and reproductive rights because of unresolved legal problems. Those go back to the start of this chapter, with Elie Mystal taking us back to the U. S. Supreme Court with this further advice:

> *You cannot be for abortion rights but against the Supreme Court's expansion anymore. The two are inextricably linked.* [18]

In the next chapter, we will explore other reasons for the poor showing of U. S. health care in comparison with that of other advanced countries.

References:

1. Mystal, E. Welcome to the juristocracy. *The Nation*, October 17-24, 2022, p. 17.
2. Richards, C. Abortion is winning issue for Harris. *New York Times*, September 20, 2024, A:23.
3. Bouie, J. Biden issues a stinging dissent. *New York Times*, August 5, 2024, p. 3.
4. Whyte, LE, Mathews, AW. CVS and Walgreens will sell abortion pills within weeks. *Wall Street Journal*, March 2-3, 2024.
5. Segars, G. Democrats are finally talking about abortion. *The New Republic*, November 2024, p. 5.
6. De Avila, J. Worry lingers as IVF restarts in Alabama. *Wall Street Journal*, March 16-17, 2024, A:3.
7. Cochrane, E. Alabama, in scramble, passes law to protect in vitro treatments. *New York Times,* March 8, 2024, A:20.
8. Littlefield, A. The abortion underground. *The Nation.* May, 2024, p. 28.
9. Miller, CC, Sanger-Katz, M. Abortions rise, even in states with rigid bans. *New York Times*, 2024, p.
10. Whyte, LE, Peterson, K, Andrews, N. RFK Jr. lays out plan to win Senate OK. *Wall Street Journal*, December 17, 2024, p. A:6.
11. Lawrence, H. *U.S. Government Publishing Office* Washington :48–804 PDF 2022 Examining The Harm To Patients From Abortion Restrictions And The Threat Of a National Abortion Ban, September 29, 2022
12. Chittister, J. As quoted by Salzillo, L. Catholic nun explains pro-life in a way that will stun many (especially Republican lawmakers). *Daily Kos*, July 30, 2015.
13. Abortion rights ballot measures win in 7 of 10 swing states. *Guttmacher Institute*, November 6, 2024.
14. Kirsinger, A, Hamel, I, Sparks, G. The role health care issues played in the 2024 election: An Analysis of AP Vote Cast.

15. Schmall, E, Maheshwari, S. Abortion groups say tech giant are suppressing posts and accounts. *New York Times*, June 12, 2024,,B:6.

16. Mackrael, K. Apple hit by first charges under EU tech law. *New York Times*, June 6, 2024, A:1.

17. Goldberg, M. Abortion bans have turned deadly. *New York Times*, September 18, 2024, A:21.

18. Liptak, A. In immunity decision, echoes of Roe v. Wade. *New York Times*, Jul 30, 2024, A:12.

Chapter 8

Increased Bureaucracy, Waste, Corruption, and Fraud

Americans will always do the right thing—after they exhaust all the alternatives.
—*Winston Churchill.* [1]

The historical accident of employer-based coverage is a huge barrier to reform. So is the way that the health insurance industry is protected in Washington by its lobbyists—five for every member of Congress. The U. S. health care system is by far the most bureaucratic and expensive system in the world, in large part because we have such an inefficient and profit-driven multi-payer financing system. In this chapter, we will describe the extent of increasing bureaucracy, waste, corruption and fraud that collectively decrease the monies available for direct patient care. Many of the references date back to the Trump 1 administration. They are retained, since they likely reflect Trump 2 starting now. Some updates are also added to reflect today's times.

I.   *Increasing Bureaucracy*

We cannot look to history for any guidance to address the problems of increasing bureaucracy in U. S. health care. The growth of managed care in the late 1980s and 1990s led to new oversized administrative bureaucracies as health maintenance organizations (HMOs) were marketed as new investor-owned for-profit companies. An ever-larger administrative bureaucracy was needed to set limits on referrals and hospitalizations, denial of services, disenrollment of sick enrollees, and such abuses as hiding performance data. Between 2000 and 2005, when the insurance market declined by one percent, its workforce grew by one-third.[2]

The Affordable Care Act increased bureaucracy further as the exchanges became consumed with such activities as determining eligibility for qualified health plans and subsidies/tax credits and verifying annual household income and family size, which are subject to change from year to year.

Administrative costs of health care in this country have increased by more than 10 percent a year since 1971. The dramatic growth in the numbers of administrators compared to physicians in the U. S. since 1970, as noted in Chapter 1, bears witness to this unparalleled growth in health care bureaucracy.

The chaos of Trumpcare insurance markets, both private and public, make the bureaucracy of health care even worse. With all the changes during Trump's first term, patients' insurance status was more volatile than ever before. Just looking at privatized Medicaid shows us what a jungle the bureaucracy had become. As one example, imagine trying to implement work requirements in the states that adopt them. Even when many thousands of Medicaid beneficiaries gain work, many of their jobs will be hourly or temporary and subject to change month by month.

As a result of this continued growth of bureaucracy in U. S. health care over these many years, physicians and their staffs are confronted with a huge time and energy burden every day that detracts from patient care and leads to increasing rates of physician burnout, especially in the more time-intensive specialties of primary care, geriatrics, and psychiatry. These are just some of the things they have to deal with before patients can be seen and treated for a primary care visit: insurance verification, pre-authorization for planned tests and procedures; determination of whether drugs will be covered by differing drug formularies among insurers; and arranging for specialist consultants after finding out their status in or out of network.

In an industry that consumes 20% of our GDP, the profiteering motive adds markedly to the work of physicians' staffs. With some 70% of physicians employed by hospitals also pushing profits, they are often working to "up-code" diagnoses that can be used for billing purposes, even when they were not involved with a given visit's care.

The differences between traditional, public Medicare and its for-profit private counterpart, Medicare Advantage, are instructive—administrative costs of Medicare Advantage are 5–6 times higher than for public Medicare.[3] Administrative costs are increased further for patients down to age 60 marketed as a public option for sale alongside private plans on the ACA's exchanges.

Agreements between health plans and participating physicians generally include a statement that the insurer has the right to determine the medical necessity of surgery, imaging studies, medication, and many other procedures. A 2017 poll by the American Medical Association concerning physician attitudes toward prior authorization found that 92 percent of respondents believe that it can have a negative impact on patient outcomes and that 84 percent find it to be a high or extremely high burden. The average time spent each week for prior authorization by physicians and their staffs was reported as 14.6 hours, or about two business days, 7 ending up with an average denial rate of about 18%. [4]

II. Waste

The growing costs of private insurance overhead and administration of insurers, physicians and other health care professionals takes both time and resources away from the main goal of the health care system—care of the patient. The overhead of the private health insurance industry in 2015 amounted to $792 per capita per year, more than five times that of Canada with its public single-payer financing system. Hospital administrative costs in the U. S. make up more than 25 percent of total hospital expenditures. Administrators in various other parts of the health care system have grown by 3,000 percent since 1970. Nurses in this country spend more than 13 hours each week to obtain prior authorizations for services, compared to none in Canada. [4]

Administrative costs are estimated to represent 25 to 31 percent of total health care expenditures in this country, twice that in Canada and considerably greater than in other OECD countries where these costs have been studied. At least 62 percent of these are for billing transactions. [6]

That 2015 study estimated that the costs of billing activities performed by primary care physicians translated to more than $99,000 per year for each primary care physician! It further estimated that the process of moving money from hospitals and physicians in the U. S. consumes some $500 billion per year, with about 80 percent of that being wasteful, including high rates of remittances that are three times higher than in other industries. CMS projected that more than $2.7 *trillion* would be spent for private health insurance overhead and administration of government health programs (mostly Medicare and Medicaid) between 2014 and 2022.

Today, with 70 percent of U. S. physicians employed by for-profit corporate employers, physicians are facing exhausting administrative burdens. Administrative spending accounts for 15-30 percent of health care spending, at least half of which is wasteful. The U. S. spends more on health care administration than comparable countries.[8] The American Medical Association has issued a statement of concern about the future supply of physicians. In view of increasing burnout of practicing physicians, the Robert Wood Johnson Foundation has begun a study about the administrative and professional burdens of medical practice, including the pressure on physicians over missed care through denials by insurers. [7, 8]

III. Corruption

Donald Trump's promise as a presidential candidate that, if elected, he would "drain the swamp" of corruption and influence peddling, has proven to be just another Trump lie. Instead, his administration in his first term was stained by unprecedented conflicts of interest that started at the top. Despite the admonitions of ethicists and the U. S. Office of Government Ethics, he refused to divest himself from his financial interests in his hotels, golf courses, restaurants, and real estate developments around the world. He just said that he would "isolate" himself from the management of the Trump Organization and put his sons in charge of the operation of the worldwide company. His businesses were reshuffled into holding companies held by a trust that Trump controlled himself. As Robert Weissman, president of Public Citizen, observed:

> *Donald Trump entered office with the most blatant and potentially corrupting conflicts of interest in the history of American politics, and things got worse from there. Business is booming at Trump International Hotel in Washington, D.C. and other Trump properties not because of the décor, but because corporations and foreign governments want to curry favor with the president.*[9]

Unabashed by his hypocrisy over ethical standards in his first term, Trump signed Executive Order 13770 one week after his inauguration titled "Ethics Commitments by Executive Branch Appointees," supposedly intended to end the revolving door between K Street and the government, including an injunction against foreign lobbying. But just six months later, the liberal super PAC found 74 lobbyists working in the administration, 49 of them in agencies they once lobbied on behalf of clients.[10] Hui Chen, former federal prosecutor who was hired as a full-time compliance expert in the Justice Department's Fraud Section in 2015, resigned six months into the Trump administration with this parting statement:

> *Trying to hold companies to standards that our current administration is not living up to was creating a cognitive dissonance that I could not overcome. . . . I am not willing to compartmentalize my values as an [ethics and compliance] professional, a citizen, and a human being... I wanted no more part [in an administration] that has so casually flouted ethics guidelines.*[11]

Despite the Executive Order, conflicts of interest and revolving door problems were pervasive in the thinly staffed first Trump administration marked by rapid turnover and ethical transgressions. Here are just three of many examples of the toxic ethical climate in his administration.

- Despite his Executive Order, Trump issued many waivers of those ethical standards, usually to individuals who had been retained by for-profit clients and then took up matters that could benefit these former clients. Larry Leggitt is one of many who received ethical waivers. He took in $400,000 as a lobbyist trying to influence Medicare policy in 2016, later becoming chief of staff in the Department of Health and Human Services in the Trump administration. [12]

- As Trump's first appointee to head the Department of Health and Human Services, Dr. Tom Price called for deep spending and staffing cuts in this department, including a $6 billion cut for the National Institutes of Health budget.[13]

- Mick Mulvaney, director of Office of Management and Budget, acknowledged that he had a hierarchy of whom he will talk to in a "pay to play" operation, with willingness to see lobbyists who had given him campaign donations but not those who did not.[14]

Today, the administrative greed of many corporate employers penetrates U. S. health care in ways that put patients at risk due to denial of essential services. One example of many is how private equity investment firms purchase of 30 hospitals in 8 states led to widespread denial of care, also involving leasing these hospitals back.[15]

IV. *Fraud*

Fraud in U. S. health care has long been a problem. Medical billing fraud, ironically enabled by electronic health records, has been estimated to account for 10 percent of all health care costs, or about $270 billion a year.[16] There are many ways how hospitals and other providers can defraud the billing process, such as disguising claims, misrepresenting operating expenses, double billing, and submitting false claims for unnecessary services or those never received by patients. Managed care plans can falsify records, collude bid-rigging, charge exorbitant "administrative fees", and withhold payments to providers or subcontractors. All this is very complicated and beyond comprehension for most of us.

Malcolm Sparrow, Professor of the Practice of Public Management at Harvard's John F. Kennedy School of Government, with ten years' experience as a detective with the British police service earlier in his career, is the leading expert in this country on health care fraud. His 1996 book, updated in 2000, *License to Steal: How Fraud Bleeds America's Health Care System*, is still the classic in the field. In 2009, Professor Sparrow gave this sobering testimony before the Subcommittee on Crime and Drugs of the Senate Committee on the Judiciary:

> *The health industry's controls are weakest with respect to outright criminal fraud. By contrast the industry's controls perform reasonably well in managing the grey and more ambiguous issues, such as questions about medical orthodoxy, pricing, and the limits of policy coverage. But criminals, who are intent on stealing as much as they can as fast as possible, and who are prepared to fabricate diagnoses, treatments, even entire medical episodes, have a relatively easy time breaking through the industry's defenses. The criminals' advantage is that they are willing to lie. And provided they learn to submit their bills correctly, they remain free to lie. The rule for criminals is simple: if you want to steal from Medicare or Medicaid, or any other health care insurance program, learn to bill your lies correctly. Then, for the most part, your claims will be paid in full and on time, without a hiccup, by a computer, and with no human involvement at all.* [17]

The following examples throughout our health care system show how pervasive fraud has been as a major problem at the expense of patients, families, and taxpayers. Unfortunately, we can expect this problem to get worse the more privatization and deregulation of health care are pursued by the incoming Trump administration, amplified as we can expect by lack of ethical standards.

Note how these examples have crossed a wide spectrum across U. S. health care:

- Federal audits of 37 private Medicare Advantage programs revealed overspending due to inflated risk scores that overstated the severity of such conditions as diabetes and depression for a majority of elderly patients treated. [18]
- An investigation by the Office of Inspector General of DHHS found widespread fraud and abuse in the Personal Care Services program of privatized Medicaid plans. [19]
- Overpayments to privatized Medicaid plans were found to be endemic in more than 30 states, often involving unnecessary or duplicative payments to providers. [20]
- Almost three-quarters of the more than 11,000 nursing homes in the country outsourced a wide variety of goods and services to companies in which they control or have a financial interest; these "related party transactions" bring higher profits to nursing homes without being recorded in their financial records even as they cut nursing staff and put patients at increased risk. [21]
- A 13-year investigation by *The Washington Post* of for-profit hospices found the industry riddled with fraud and abuse, commonly seeking out less sick patients who need less care and live longer, yielding higher profits, and even encouraging their employees to recruit such patients. [22]
- Medical identity theft has been found whereby criminals steal personal data from millions of Americans to get health care, prescriptions and medical equipment; this can result in victims having claims denied, losing insurance coverage, and/ or adverse impacts on their credit ratings.

This is how Ralph Nader has summed up the economic and political challenges in dealing with health care fraud:

> *All in all, the health care industry is replete with rackets that neither honest practitioners or regulators find worrisome enough to effectively challenge. The perverse economic incentives in this industry range from third party payments to third party procedures. Add paid-off members of Congress who starve enforcement budgets and the enormous profits that come from that tired triad 'waste, fraud and abuse' and you have a massive problem needing a massive solution.* [23]

Concluding comment

Unfortunately, as we have just embarked on the second Trump administration under Project 2025, the problems discussed in this chapter will only get worse, especially with unqualified appointees trying to manage this large part of the economy.

There is a fix, however, to what has become a long-term massive problem of escalating bureaucracy, waste, corruption and fraud driven by greed in an increasingly unaccountable corporatized "system". Single-payer financing, with everyone having a national health insurance card, would eliminate most of this while saving more than $600 billion a year through simplified administration, negotiated fees for health professionals, global budgets for hospitals and other facilities, and transition toward a not-for-profit service-oriented system. We will discuss all that in Chapter 12. But for now, let's move to the next chapter where we will see that deregulation in the Trump administration is one more reason that today's health care policies will not work, are detrimental to the public interest, and are unsustainable.

References:

1. Churchill. The Churchill Documents, November 1895, *The Churchill Project*. Hillsdale College.

2. Krugman, P. The world of U. S. health care economics is downright scary. *Seattle Post Intelligencer*, September 26, 2006: B1.

3. AMA. 2017 AMA Prior Authorization Physician Survey, December 2017.

4. MGMA. *Pole*, May 16, 2017

5. Himmelstein, DU, Woolhandler, S. The post-launch problem: The Affordable Care Act's persistently high administrative costs. *Health Affairs Blog*, May 27, 2015.

6. Tseng, Administrative costs associated with physician billing.

7. Carey, L. Rural communities face primary care physician shortage. *The Progressive Populist*, June 1, 2024, p. 1.)

8. PNHP launches Moral Injury Project. *PNHP Fall Newsletter*, 2024.

9. Weisman, R, as quoted by Zibel, A. Presidency for sale. *Public Citizen News*, March/April 2018, pp. 8-9.

10. Nazaryan, A. The swamp runneth over. *Newsweek*, November 10, 2017.

11. Johnson, J. Top ethics official resigns, says working for Trump requires 'abandonment of conscience'. *Common Dreams*, July 3, 2017.

12. Rmuse, Opinion: Swindler Trump is using the White House to rip off taxpayers. *PoliticusUSA*, March 21, 2017.

13. Lipton, E, Ivory, D. Lobbyists, industry lawyers were granted ethics waivers to work in Trump Administration. *New York Times*, June 8, 2017

14. Markay, L, Stein, S. Mick Mulvaney met with lobbyist donors while at Trump White House. *Daily Beast*, April 27, 2018.

15. Brownstein, M. Private equity's appetite for hospitals may put patients at risk. *Harvard T. H. Chan School of Public Health*, December 16, 2024.

16. Buchheit, P. Private health care as an act of terrorism. *Common Dreams*, July 20, 2015: 1.

17. Sparrow, MK. Testimony before Senate Committee on the Judiciary, Subcommittee on Crime and Drugs. *Criminal Prosecution as a Deterrent to Health Care Fraud*. May 20, 2009.

18. Schulte, F. Audits of some Medicare Advantage plans reveal pervasive overcharging. *NPR Now* KPLU, August 29, 2016.

19. Bailey, M. Seniors suffer amid widespread fraud by Medicaid caretakers. *Kaiser Health News*, November 7, 2016.

20. Herman, B. Medicaid's unmanaged managed care. *Modern Healthcare*, April 30, 2016.

21. Rau, J. Care suffers as more nursing homes feed money into corporate webs. *Kaiser Health News*, December 31, 2017.

22. McCauley, L. Investigation reveals rampant fraud by privatized hospice groups. *Common Dreams*, December 17, 2013.

23. Nader, R. In the public interest. Follow the hospital bills. *The Progressive Populist* 18 (4): 19, March 1, 2012.

Chapter 9

Deregulation Of Health Care

A constant mantra during Trump's campaign and during his first term was to claim that we are over-regulated. It was assumed that deregulation of health, safety, labor, financial, and environmental sectors would somehow get us on a better track in this country. His simplistic policy seems to be that regulations are bad, will take away jobs, and deregulation will improve the economy. In his first term he issued an executive order ten days after taking office that government agencies should kill two rules for every new one they propose.

Trump's Cabinet was loyal to the cause and took on the "deconstruction of the administrative state." This new direction toward small government had the strong support of the Freedom Caucus (including House Tea Party members), many trade organizations (including the Chamber of Commerce and the National Association of Manufacturers), and corporate lobbyists. [1]

This chapter has two goals: (1) to describe the kinds of deregulatory actions that have been taken across various parts of the health care system; and (2) to ask and try to answer whether U.S. health care can be regulated in the public, not corporate interest?

I. Deregulation Across the Health Care System

Let's look at how the emphasis on deregulation in recent years, accelerated during the first Trump administration, has played out in eight parts of our health care system.

1. Insurance industry

Regulation of private health insurance has always been lax. For many years, most regulatory authority has been given to the states, where the insurance lobby dominates state capitols.

Insurance regulators in the states have long had a cozy relationship with industry. As one example, the Center for Public Integrity has found that one-half of state insurance commissioners who have left their jobs in the last ten years have gone to work for the industry they were supposedly regulating. [2]

The ACA continued that trend, with minimal federal oversight over states. Now there is even less federal oversight, with big variations from one state to another. As we have seen in earlier chapters, states now have even more leeway under Trumpcare. The DHHS permits marketing of plans that do not comply with the ACA's regulations, which require coverage of all ten essential health benefits, banning of annual and lifetime limits, and not setting premiums based on age, health status and history. Meanwhile, with little public scrutiny, private insurers are vacuuming up personal details of hundreds of Americans which can be used to raise premiums or deny coverage.[3]

2. Hospital industry

In contrast to the insurance industry, the hospital industry is over-regulated, but much of the regulatory process is fundamentally flawed. A recent report from the American Hospital Association describes the complexity and inefficiencies of this process. Health systems, hospitals, and post-acute providers, such as long-term care hospitals and skilled nursing facilities, must comply with 629 discrete regulatory requirements across nine domains. These requirements are promulgated by four different federal agencies and are often duplicative. They must also comply with many stringent contract requirements imposed by payers, such as private Medicare and Medicaid plans and commercial payers. An average-size hospital employs 59 full-time people, more than one-quarter of whom are doctors and nurses, to stay in compliance.[4]

Despite this immense effort to comply with federal regulations, the burdensome process fails to meet the goal of best protecting the public. Most hospitals are accredited by a Joint Commission with a board mostly composed of executives of health systems it accredits as well as members named by health care lobbying groups. Most hospitals that are found to have safety violations keep their full 'Gold Seal of Approval.'[5] Their track record, however, has big problems.

A 2016 study of 22 million hospital admissions found that patients are 3 times more likely to die in the worst hospitals and 13 times more likely to have medical complications compared to the best hospitals. [6]

3. Surgery centers

Surgery centers started almost 50 years ago as low-cost alternatives for minor surgical procedures. Since then, their numbers have soared to more than 5,600 in the U. S., and they have become a hazard for many patients. A 2007 report by Medicare noted that "surgery centers have neither patient safety standards consistent with those in hospitals, nor are they required to have the trained staff and equipment needed to provide the breadth of intensity of care . . . Some procedures are unsafe to be handled at surgery centers." [7]

These problems call for more regulation of surgery centers:

- Surgery centers take on many major surgical procedures, including complex spinal surgeries.
- More than 260 patients have died since 2013 after in-and-out care at U. S. surgery centers, many as a result of inadequate treatment of complications; it is not uncommon for staff to call 911 in these instances.
- At least 7,000 patients required transfer to a hospital in the year that ended in September 2017. [8]

4. Drug industry

The drug industry has effectively lobbied over many years to avoid price controls and other regulations over its promotion and marketing practices. Since 1993, it has managed a big effort through direct-to-consumer drug advertising, banned in many advanced countries, often with misinformation and false claims. The industry brought out a new argument in 2017 based on the First Amendment in an attempt to evade drug safety rules and sell more medications for off-label marketing of unapproved drugs. [9]

The industry has long lobbied against importation of drugs from other countries and for faster action by the FDA for approvals with less rigorous oversight. Since 1962, the previous gold standard for FDA approval required "substantial evidence" of a drug's efficacy based on controlled clinical trials. The passage of the 21st Century Cures Act drastically lowered the standards for FDA approval of new drugs to a new "standard" based on "real world evidence" (read non-rigorous uncontrolled observational data easily gamed by drug manufacturers through their marketing departments).[10] The FDA itself is plagued by underfunding, lack of sufficient authority, and conflicts of interest. The industry supports much of the FDA's budget through user fees.[11]

Corporate greed trumps patient safety through this lax regulatory process. As just one of many examples, a study of FDA-approved drugs subsequently withdrawn from the market between 1993 and 2010 found that unsafe drugs were prescribed more than 100 million times in the U. S. before being recalled from the market.[12]

5. Medical device industry

The medical device industry is larger than most of us might think, with an enormous market ranging from cardiac pacemakers and defibrillators to lasers, hip and knee replacements. Also regulated by the FDA, this industry follows the same pattern as the drug industry, putting profits ahead of patient safety.[13] Medical device manufacturers often delay notification to the FDA about negative experiences with their products, continue marketing them beyond adverse reports, and seek support from willing legislators. Johnson & Johnson's defective all-metal ASR hip replacement is one example of this delaying action, which ended up in the filing of some 5,000 lawsuits against the company. [14]

6. Nursing homes

Nursing homes have never been regulated in the public interest. Two-thirds of them are for-profit, placing profits ahead of service. Compared to not-for-profit nursing homes, for-profit chains are typically investor owned, have lower staffing levels, worse quality of care, and higher death rates. A report by the Inspector General 2012 found that for-profit nursing homes overbilled Medicare by $1.5 billion a year for treatments that patients didn't need and never received. [15]

The first Trump administration rolled back many of the previous regulations on nursing homes. In February 2018, the administration imposed an 18-month moratorium on imposing fines or denials of federal payments when nursing homes fail to meet certain requirements, such as ensuring that they have adequate staffing or are using psychotropic drugs correctly.[16] In opposition to this moratorium, a group of Democratic senators, led by Sen. Richard Blumenthal (D-CT) and Sen. Amy Klobuchar (D-MN), sent a letter to Alex Azar at DHHS, voicing serious concern that "this will inevitably weaken the safety of our nation's nursing homes and put patients, many of whom are elderly and wholly reliant on this care, at greater risk." [17]

7. Hospices

Two-thirds of the nation's hospices are for-profit. Compared to their not-for profit counterparts, for-profits offer fewer services and provide worse quality of care.[18] The number of for-profit hospices almost doubled from 2000 to 2013, with Medicare spending for that care going up by five-fold. As we saw in the last chapter, the industry is riddled with fraud and abuse. [19]

8. Laboratory tests

There is a large under recognized multi-billion-dollar-a-year business in "lab-developed tests" that is virtually unregulated. These tests have rarely been scrutinized by the FDA, gone through clinical trials, or been proven accurate or medically useful before going to market. As the adverse impacts of inaccurate tests have become widespread, the FDA is now trying to better regulate this industry, seeing these tests as the Wild West of medicine. Examples of tests with unproven effectiveness include the BRCA gene test for breast cancer, which has led some women to undergo bilateral mastectomies unnecessarily, and a KIF6 gene test as a way to detect a predisposition to heart disease. A study of 55 cancer-care and testing websites by researchers at Harvard and the Dana-Farber Cancer Center concluded that "most of the websites have little or no evidence substantiating the ability to improve patient outcome." [20]

II. Can Health Care Be Regulated in the Public Interest?

As is obvious from the foregoing, we have a poor track record in this country in trying to regulate the health care industry in the public interest. A major obstacle is the use of big corporate money to lobby for deregulation in Congress, as represented by the green wave of dark money. The regulatory process is lax or far too complex, ineffective, and hijacked by corporate stakeholders protecting their prerogatives in a free-wheeling market-based system. Health care is being treated as just another commodity for sale on an open market that is oriented to increasing corporate revenues at the expense of patient care. Figure 9.1 illustrates the ongoing political bribery through large corporate lobbying and campaign donations that have been so persistent in limiting regulation over these many years. This failure leads us to question how and whether we can achieve regulatory protection of patient safety.

Figure 9.1

THE GREEN WAVE OF DARK MONEY

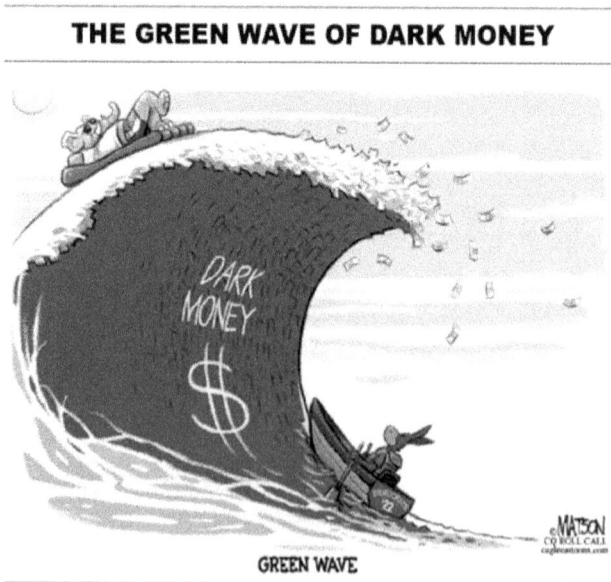

Source: *Matson Roll Call*. Reprinted with permission

The idea that markets will self-correct has been proven wrong over many years. This situation is all the more challenging because of GOP control of Congress and the Trump administration, ideologically opposed as they are to more regulation and in favor of smaller government. The first Trump administration launched a deregulatory bonanza. As one example, penalties for corporate crime and misconduct of the country's 100 most profitable corporations dropped from about $17 billion a year during the Obama administration to just $1.1 billion in Trump's first year in office. [21]

The appointment of Lina Khan to head up the FDA during the Biden administration made an excellent start toward restoring stronger regulatory oversight of U. S. health care. Her tenure has been forceful and very much needed and is a good start toward further progress. [22] Unfortunately, however, she was fired at the start of the second Trump administration. A larger role of government will continue to be essential if we are to achieve significant correction of unethical and profit-driven practices within the medical-industrial complex that put patients at risk.

We need to come to grips with the concept that the goal of our health care should be to best advance the interests of patients, not corporate earnings, as so many other advanced countries around the world have done for years. The common good should be at the heart of health policy, which can never happen within the present culture of health care. As John Adams, the second president of the United States and one of our founding fathers, said:

> *Government is instituted for the common good: for the protection, safety, prosperity and happiness of the people;—and not for the profit, honor, or private interest of any one man, family, or class of men.* [24]

The ACA introduced new supposedly "value-based" initiatives that theoretically might improve the quality of patient care, such as pay-for-performance" (P4P) report cards for physicians and accountable care organizations. Although we now have some 150 quality metrics in use for evaluating outpatient services, there is still no evidence that any of them improve care. Instead, aided by electronic health records that have largely become billing instruments, they consume much of physicians' and their staffs' time and are easily gamed by up-coding for maximal revenue, usually to physicians' employers.[23,24]

We know that up to one-third of all health care services provided are inappropriate, unnecessary, and even dangerous to patients in some instances. But they are the result of a system based on maximal profits, not the best interests of patients.

In order to rein in the excesses of today's profit-driven health care system, we will need financing reform. The regulatory burden now being placed on health systems, hospitals, and post-acute care providers that require regular reporting across nine domains, leads Dr. Don McCanne, senior health policy fellow and past president of Physicians for a National Health Program, to say:

> *A quick look at the nine domains of regulatory overload is all you need to be reminded of the nightmare created by these evolving requirements. Inefficiencies, wasted resources, and provider burnout ensue, which negatively impact the primary mission of the health care system: patient care. . . Think of the recoverable administrative waste that characterizes our fragmented health care financing system—most of which is in the private sector. We spend over a trillion dollars a year on administration, and somewhere around $300 billion to $500 billion is recoverable merely by transitioning to a well-designed single payer system.* [25]

Fast forward to the pre-inaugural days before Trump's second term, and we had an even more destructive phase of the regulatory process. Elon Musk, the richest man in the world and owner of Twitter with all its disinformation, took on a "co-president" role with Trump. He was accountable to nobody as Director of the Department of Government Efficiency. His conflicts of interest included having bought his way to this role and harboring various sources of ongoing governmental contracts. In that capacity, he was planning cutbacks in government funding by some $2-$4 trillion without any knowledge of what these cuts would mean to health care. Combine that with the complexity of U. S. health care described, and you had a perfect storm. [26] As this book goes to press, he has left government to return to his private businesses. It is unclear how much money he actually saved the government.

Concluding comment

Given that Trumpcare involves far less regulation than will be required to protect patients, it is time to move on to the next three chapters where we will describe the various ways that Trumpcare is failing, but also open-up new opportunities to reform U. S. health care in the public interest.

References:

1. Steinzor, R. The war on regulation. *The American Prospect*, Spring 2017, pp. 72-76.
2. Mishak, MJ. Drinks, junkets and jobs. How the insurance industry courts state commissioners. *The Washington Post*, October 2, 2016.
3. Allen, M. Health insurers are vacuuming up details about you—and it may raise your rates. *ProPublica*, July 17, 2018.
4. Regulatory overload: Assessing the regulatory burden on health systems, hospitals, and post-acute care providers. *American Hospital Association*, October 2017.
5. Armour, S. Hospitals keep 'gold seal' despite woes. *Wall Street Journal*, September 9-10: A1, 2017.
6. Abelson, R. Go to the wrong hospital and you're 3 times more likely to die. *New York Times*, December 4, 2016.
7. Jewett, C, Alesia, M. Surgery centers boom, patients are paying with their lives. Kaiser Health News and USA TODAY Network, March 2, 2018.
8. Ibid # 7.
9. Feng, R. PhRMA's latest excuse for off-label marketing won't fly. *Public Citizen* 37 (1): Jan/Feb 2017, p. 1.
10. Gaffney, A. Congress just quietly handed drug companies a dangerous victory. New Republic, December 14, 2016.
11. Demko, P. Healthcare's hired hands: When the stakes rise in Washington,

healthcare interests seek well-connected lobbying firms. *Modern Health- care*, October 6, 2014.

12. Saluja, S, Woolhandler, S, Himmelstein, DU et al. Unsafe drugs were pre- scribed more than one hundred million times in the United States before being recalled. *Intl J Health Services*, June 14, 2016.

13. Burton, TM. FDA faulted over medical devices. *Wall Street Journal*, Sep- tember 30, 2014.

14. Meier, B. Hip implants U. S. rejected sold overseas. New York Times, Feb- ruary 12, 2012: A1.

15. Waldman, P. For-profit nursing homes lead in overcharging while care suffers. *Bloomberg Business*, December 31, 2012.

16. Press release. Department of Justice, October 24, 2016.

17. Weixel, N. Dems seek reversal of nursing home regulatory rollback. *The Hill*, February 20, 2018.

18. Perry, J, Stone, R. In the business of dying: Questioning the commercial- ization of hospice. J Law, Medicine, and Ethics, May 18, 2011.

19. McCauley, L. Investigation reveals rampant fraud by privatized hospice groups. *Common Dreams*, December 17, 2013.

20. Burton, TM. The 'wild west' of medicine. *Wall Street Journal*, December 11, 2015: A1.

21. Johnson, J. Tracking tool shows fines for corporate misconduct have plum- meted under Trump. *Common Dreams*, February 13, 2018.

22. Smith, TJ. F.T.C. chief's time may be up. Her tenure has been forceful. *New York Times,* September 30, 2024, B:3.

23. Casalino, LP, Gans, , Weber, R et al. U. S. physician practices spend more than $15.4 billion annually to report quality measures. *Health Affairs*, March 2016.

24. Meinrath, SD. AI and the quest for eternal vigilance. *The Progressive,* October-November 2024, pp. 8-9.

25. McCanne, D. Comment on Ibid # 4. The cost of regulatory overload. Quote of the Day, October 27, 2017.

26. Reich, R. Musk's dangerous bullying. *The Progressive Populist*, January 1-15, 2025.

Chapter 10

Inadequate Oversight and Accountability

*So it is that contrary to what we have heard
rhetorically for a generation now, the individualist, greed-
driven, free-market ideology is at odds with our history
and with what most Americans really care about. More
and more people agree that growing inequality is bad for
the country, that corporations have too much power, that
money in politics is corrupting democracy and that working
families and poor communities need and deserve help
when the market system fails to generate shared prosperity.
Indeed, the American public is committed to a set of
values that almost perfectly contradicts the conservative
agenda that has dominated politics for a generation now.*

—Bill Moyers, leading journalist, political
commentator, and Television Hall of Famer [1]

The last six chapters have described how Trumpcare is bound
to fail the public interest and common good while benefitting
corporate stakeholders at the expense of everyday Americans.
We have already seen how privatization and deregulation in our
market-based system go hand in hand and do not assure access to
affordable health care of acceptable quality.

This chapter adds one more reason for Trumpcare's inevitable
failure—the increasingly inadequate mechanisms for oversight
and accountability of health care. This has been recognized by Bill
Moyers as a long-term problem, but it is all the worse under the
Trump administration.

This chapter has three goals: (1) to briefly consider the
problems of accountability of our present multi-payer financing

vs. that of a single-payer financing system; (2) to give examples that illustrate how the lack of oversight and accountability of health care has been so widespread across our non-system; and (3) to discuss the necessary and appropriate role of government in ensuring adequate quality and safety of health care in this country.

I.   *Goals for Multi-Payer vs. Single-Payer Health Care*

Periodic international studies of health care systems in high income countries have long found that the U. S. still fails to have established goals for health care for overall accountability. Donald Light, Ph.D., Professor of Social and Behavioral Medicine at the University of Dentistry of New Jersey, recommended these appropriate goals more than 20 years ago:

1. Everyone is covered, and everyone contributes in proportion to his or her income.
2. Decisions about all matters are open and publicly debated. Accountability for costs, quality, and value of providers, suppliers, and administrators is public.
3. Contributions do not discriminate by type of illness or ability to pay.
4. Coverage does not discriminate by type of illness or ability to pay.
5. Coverage responds first to medical need and suffering.
6. Non-financial barriers by class, language, education, and geography are to be minimized.
7. Providers are paid fairly and equitably, taking into account their local circumstances.
8. Clinical waste is minimized through self-care, prevention, strong primary care, and identification of unnecessary procedures.
9. Financial waste is minimized through simplified administrative arrangements and strong bargaining for good value.
10. Choice is maximized in a common playing field where 90-95 percent of payments go toward necessary and efficient health services and only 5-10 percent toward administration.[2]

Despite the obvious logic to these recommendations, however, the U. S. has consistently failed to adopt such an approach for universal health care for all. Our huge health care industry, 20% of our gross national product, continues on with corporatized employer health insurance that knows no bounds for cost or quality control. These circumstances led Wendell Potter to this conclusion during the COVID pandemic:

> *America needs to get out of the business linking health insurance to job status. Even in better times, this arrangement was a bad idea from a health perspective. Most Americans whose families depend on their employers for coverage are just a layoff from being uninsured. And now, when many businesses are shutting down and considering layoffs, it's a public health disaster.*[3]

II. *Deteriorating Accountability under Trumpcare*

These are some of the many ways that the Trump administration has avoided accountability of health care:

1. Lower FDA standards

The Federal Drug Administration (FDA) dates back more than 100 years. It has an enormous job, bearing responsibility for the safety and efficacy of all human and veterinary drugs, biologic products, medical devices, and products emitting radiation that are sold in the U. S. User fees from the drug industry that it regulates make up a large part of its budget, so that the FDA is to a considerable extent held hostage by that industry. As a result, there are many ongoing conflicts of interest in its advisory committees and other parts of the approval process.

As it pushes for faster approval of its drugs on weaker evidence, the drug industry has successfully opposed the use of cost-effectiveness as a criterion for drug or device approval or requiring new drug applications to demonstrate benefit over competitor drugs, not just placebo. The FDA increasingly approves new drugs based on lower standards of evidence, then requires post-approval studies to further assess safety and efficacy. Unfortunately, the FDA is typically underfunded and lacks regulatory teeth.

2.   *Pharmaceutical industry*

As we saw in Chapter 2, the drug industry has effectively lobbied the government for many years to retain its ability to set drug prices and avoid price controls. Drug manufacturers set prices to whatever the market will bear as they lobby government to spread its influence in Washington, D. C. As just one example, Novo Nordisk, which produces Levemir, a long-acting insulin, runs its own political action committee (PAC) and has asked more than 400 of its employees to contact lawmakers and their staffs on Capitol Hill. It raised the wholesale price of a vial of Levimir from $144.80 in 2012 to $335.70 in 2018, and was under investigation by state attorneys general for predatory pricing. [4]

Meanwhile, of course, drug prices keep going up. Over the five years since 2013, prices for the top 20 drugs prescribed for older Americans rose by an average of 12 percent a year, with seven of those drugs increasing by more than 100 percent. [5]

3. *Drug Enforcement Agency (DEA) and opioids*

The use of *prescribed* opioids, such as hydrocodone and oxycodone, has soared over the last 20 years, led by a multi-faceted campaign underwritten by the pharmaceutical industry that touted the use of these drugs for chronic pain with little chance of addiction. That led to an epidemic that killed more than 200,000 Americans, more than three times the number of U. S. military deaths in the Vietnam War. Initially, Joe Rannazzisi of the DEA stood tall in enforcement actions against wholesale drug distributors that were shipping huge volumes of prescription opioids to targeted corrupt physicians and pharmacists engaged in a very lucrative black market.

A powerful backlash from industry, however, soon began to neutralize the DEA through recruitment by the pharmaceutical industry of at least 56 DEA and DOJ officials and PAC committees calling for legislative action. Spearheaded by Rep. Tom Marino (R-PA), the result was the passage of the disingenuously named

Ensuring Patient Access and Effective Drug Enforcement Act of 2016 that raised the bar for enforcement to a "higher standard", from "an imminent danger to the community" to "a substantial likelihood of an imminent threat." That law made it almost impossible for the DEA to freeze suspicious shipments of hundreds of millions of opioid pills from wholesalers, and the number of enforcement actions by the DEA dropped precipitously. Rannazzisi was forced out of the DEA in 2015, then Trump nominated Marino to head up the Office of National Drug Control Policy until his name was withdrawn after his role in defanging the DEA was exposed by an investigative report by *The Washington Post* and *CBS 60 Minutes*. Since then, lawsuits have been filed in federal court in five states bringing claims of fraud and racketeering as well as unjust profits made by defendant companies. [6]

4. Private health insurers

The Trump administration has promised short-term insurance plans that offer lower premiums, "more choice", and much less coverage in getting around the ACA's requirement to cover ten essential benefits. The big tradeoff is lower premiums for less protection for healthy people, to the extent that these plans hardly qualify as insurance. A recent study by the Kaiser Family Foundation of short-term policies in 45 states plus the District of Columbia found that none covered maternity care, 71 percent excluded outpatient prescription drugs, 62 percent do not cover substance abuse disorders, and 43 percent don't cover mental health services. The cheapest plans have very high deductibles and other cost sharing exceeding $20,000. [7]

Short-term plans still exacerbate two public health crises—the worst rate of maternal deaths in the developed world and the deadliest drug epidemic in U. S. history. They also destabilize the risk pool for health insurance, attracting healthier people, avoiding those with such "deniable" conditions as diabetes, cancer, pregnancy, or HIV/AIDS, and raising premiums for older, sicker people to an unaffordable extent. More insurers are complaining of shrinking markets and a "death spiral" for the private health insurance industry.

5. Privatized Medicare and Medicaid

As we saw in Chapter 5, privatization of both of these essential programs leads to gaming the reimbursement system for higher profits, long waiting times, worse care, and often fraud. As a result, taxpayers and the government pay more and get less with little oversight or accountability.

6. Payment abuses

Today's reimbursement system with multiple payers has led to widespread abuses in payments to physicians and other health professionals. California gives us insight into what is going on. Despite passage of a state law in 2000 intended to rein in payment abuses by health care service plans, a recent survey reported these findings:

• Two-thirds of physician respondents had routine problems with unfair payment practices, such as repeated delays in adjudication and correct reimbursement of their claims.

• More than one-half of the physician practices reported that health plans attempted to rescind or modify authorizations after physicians had provided the services in good faith.

• Resolution processes were largely ineffective.

• Anthem and Blue Shield of California had the most unfair payment practices.

• Statewide, the Department of Managed Health Care has taken few enforcement actions against plans that engage in unfair payment practices. [8]

7. Nursing homes

Nursing homes across the country have serious safety and accountability problems. Infection control is routinely ignored. At the same time, the Trump administration scaled back the use of penalties to punish nursing homes that violate standards that put residents at risk of injury. Part of the problem is the practice of three-quarters of U. S. nursing homes, in their pursuit of higher profits, to outsource services to companies that they control or in which they have an interest. Commonly owned companies are more likely to engage in and conceal fraud while having higher rates of patient injury than their not-for-profit counterparts.[9] Discharges and evictions have become a top-ranking category of grievances among nursing home residents, especially when their Medicare coverage reaches its limits. [10]

8. Assisted living

According to a 2018 report by the Government Accountability Office, many billions of dollars of government spending are going to deregulated assisted living facilities that operate under a patchwork of vague standards and limited oversight by state and federal authorities. The care of hundreds of thousands of patients, especially Medicaid beneficiaries, is jeopardized in these facilities, where elder abuse is widespread, including physical, emotional, and sexual abuse of residents. [11]

9. Prisons: non-payment of court fines and mental illness

As we saw in Chapter 5 for-profit private prisons have become a huge industry that operates below the radar with little accountability. As Trump and Republican legislators were celebrating their December 2017 historic tax-cut (mostly for the wealthy), Trump's appointee as Attorney General reinstated a draconian policy that targets the poor—a return to the equivalent of debtors' prisons. They were banned in the U. S. in 1833 and the Supreme Court has affirmed on three different occasions in the last century that the 14th Amendment prohibits incarceration for non-payment of exorbitant court-imposed fines or fees. Unfortunately, many cities have grown to rely on these fines and fees as a major source of revenue. [12]

Many more people with mental illness are housed across the U. S. in jails than in psychiatric hospitals. This is a major problem, since those in jails have poor access to psychiatric care. There tends to be insufficient staff training to deal with the mentally ill, to the extent that inmate suicides, self-mutilation and violence frequently result. [13]

10. *Dismantling of the Environmental Protection Agency (EPA)*

The EPA has been charged with safeguarding our air, water, land and climate from corporate polluters for almost 50 years. Scott Pruitt was Trump's appointee in his first term to head the EPA. When he was Oklahoma's Attorney General, he sued the EPA at least 14 times to block clean air and water standards at the bidding of fossil fuel companies and other big polluters. An example of Pruitt's attack on the EPA's original role: he granted a "financial hardship" waiver to billionaire investor Carl Icahn, who reported a net income of $234.4 million in 2014. [14] Robert Redford, longtime Board Member of the National Resources Defense Council (NRDC), summons up the serious concerns this way:

> *Administrator Pruitt is tearing down environmental safeguards while putting his agency at the beck and call of industries that exist to pollute and profit. You can be sure the rest of us will pay the price—in deadly smog, undrinkable water, devastated wildlands, and a drastically warming climate.* [15]

III. *Role of Government in Ensuring Accountability of Health Care*

It is time to admit that an unfettered market-based system with little real competition and increasing consolidation by corporate giants will never lead to a health care system that serves the common good. Obama's ACA made some progress in expanding the number of Americans with health insurance, but there are still more than 30 million uninsured, tens of millions underinsured, and cost containment is nowhere in sight. This is how an overview assessment in *The Lancet*, a leading medical journal in the U. K., sees our situation:

What Americans got with the Affordable Care Act was complicated insurance marketplaces in every state with a complex array of confusing private insurance products. The health reform process was exposed, in the words of the British medical journal The Lancet, "How corporate influence renders the U. S. government incapable of making policy on the basis of evidence and the public interest." [16]

Dr. Marcia Angell, former editor of *The New England Journal of Medicine* and author of *The Truth About Drug Companies: How They Deceive Us and What We Can Do About It*, brings us this important insight:

The fatal flaw in Obamacare is that it is inherently unsustainable. (Unfortunately, the Republicans are right that it is unraveling, but wrong about the reason, and certainly wrong that the solution is more market competition.) Obama made the mistake of trying to increase access to better health insurance without fundamentally altering the features of our health system that made it so expensive, inflationary, and inadequate in the first place. Thus he continued to rely on investor-owned insurance companies and even guaranteed them millions more customers, while he also relied on revenue-seeking providers, including hospital conglomerates (even if technically nonprofit), out-patient facilities, drug companies, and medical specialists paid to provide ever more and ever pricier tests and procedures... The result is that we still don't have a health care system. Rather, we have a non-system, consisting of thousands of businesses operating more or less independently of one another, each seeking to expand revenues and profits, often by avoiding uninsured or otherwise costly patients. [17]

Trumpcare has made access to affordable health care progressively worse. Increasing privatization, further deregulation, and shifting responsibility for health care to the states all work to increase waste and bureaucracy as the nation's safety net unravels further. Our present health care policies fail the public interest and benefit corporate stakeholders at the expense of patients, their families, and taxpayers. The prognosis for our non-system is poor unless we can acknowledge failure of our present directions and adopt fundamental reforms to be described in Chapter 12. Otherwise we can expect budget cuts and federal waivers to states, uncontrolled health care prices, and growing numbers of preventable early deaths due to the high costs of drugs and the lack of insurance coverage.

If we are to improve and reform our system, we need more government involvement in health care instead of less. The following are areas where federal government oversight is critical, with health policy based on experience and evidence, protected from corporate influence and lobbyists:

1. Establish and protect universal access to affordable health care for all through single-payer Medicare for All.
2. Price controls, including negotiated prices of drugs and medical devices.
3. Global budgets for hospitals and other facilities; negotiated fees for physicians and other health professionals.
4. Planning for new facilities based on population needs for adequate access.
5. Workforce planning, to include goals to rebuild shortage fields, especially in primary care, psychiatry, and geriatrics; revision of present graduation medical education financing policies to support these goals.
6. Strengthen the authority of such federal agencies as the FDA and DEA, including adequate funding and protection from political influence.
7. Establish a national agency for science-based evaluation of treatments, based on efficacy and cost-effectiveness, free from conflicts of interest with industry.
8. Adopt policies intended to limit health care disparities, support equity, and reinforce a service ethic in health care.

Concluding comment

You can't deregulate a failing health care system if you want to improve and reform it in the public interest. There are stark differences between Trumpcare and GOP health care proposals and needed reforms in the public interest. The results will be bad if GOP policies are not blocked by progressive Democrats in coming election cycles. In the last chapter, we will discuss how we can finally get health care reform right.

References:

1. Moyers, B. A new story for America. *The Nation* 284 (3):17, 2007.
2. Light, DW. A conservative call for universal access to health care. Penn Bioeth J, 9 (4): 4-6, 2002.
3. Potter, W., healthcare uncovered@substack.com, Dec. 9, 2024
4. Hancock, J, Lucas, E. How a drug company under pressure for high prices ratchets up political activity. *Kaiser Health News*, April 30, 2018.
5. Wapner, J. Pharmapocalypse. *Newsweek.com*, May 4, 2018.
6. Geyman, JP. The opioid epidemic: fueled by greed, corruption, and complicit government. *Daily Kos* and others, October 19, 2017.
7. Randazzo, S. New front in opioid lawsuits: rise in insurance premiums. *Wall Street Journal*, May 3, 2018.
8. Pollitz, K. Yes, the Trump administration promotes consumer choice—for healthy people. *The Washington Post*, May 1, 2018.
9. California Medical Association. CMA survey finds rampant health plan payment abuses. April 2, 2018.
10. Gorman, A. Weak oversight blamed for poor care at California nursing homes going unchecked. *Kaiser Health News*, May 4, 2018.
11. Bernard, TS, Pear, R. Complaints about nursing home evictions rise, and regulators take note. *New York Times*, February 22, 2018.
12. Pear, R. U. S. pays billions for 'assisted living,' but what does it get? *New York Times*, February 3, 2018.
13. Tesfaye, S. A return to debtors' prisons: Jeff Sessions' war on the poor. *Truthout*, December 31, 2017.

14. Gorman, A. Use of psychiatric drugs soars in California jails. *Kaiser Health News*, May 8, 2018.

15. Redford, R. New York. *NRDC*, April, 2018.

16. Ansell, DA, *The Death Gap: How Inequality Kills.* Chicago and London. *University of Chicago Press*, 2017, p. 137; quoting *The Lancet* 374, December 5, 2009.

17. Angell, M. Single payer: the single path. *Democracy. A Journal of Ideas.* Winter 2017.

PART IV

TOWARD A BRIGHT FUTURE WITH NATIONAL HEALTH INSURANCE

The idea of a common good was once widely understood and accepted in America. After all, the U. S. Constitution was designed for 'We the people' seeking to 'promote the general welfare'—not for 'me the narcissist' seeking as much wealth and power as possible.

. . . If we're losing our national identity, it's not because we now come in more colors, practice more religions, and speak more languages than we once did. It is because we are forgetting the real meaning of America— the ideals on which our nation was built. We are losing our sense of the common good. [1]

—Robert B. Reich, professor of public policy at the University of California, Berkeley, chairman of Common Cause, and author of the new book, *The Common Good*

"I just want to be dictator for one day" [2]
—Donald J. Trump in January 2025.

Lo and behold, the entity that becomes the most persistent in alleging that American elections are fraudulent, fake, rigged, and everything else turns out to be the President of the United States. [3]

—Anne Applebaum, staff writer at *The Atlantic* and author of the new book, *Autocracy, Inc.: The Dictators Who Want to Rule the World*

Right in front of our eyes, you're seeing the destruction of the United States of America, and the beginning of a dictatorship run by a career criminal and his enablers drawn from the worst among us. [4]

—David Cay Johnston, February 11, 2025, *DCR Report*

These are the polar-opposites, which divide the choices that were made by the 2024 U.S. presidential election. A choice was made between a well-tested servant of government and a convicted felon telling us, through consistent lies, that he will be an autocrat all the way, if elected. The devious nature of the takeover of our health care system is laid out, together with elimination of non-Trump loyalists in government, in the Heritage Foundation's *Project 2025 Mandate for Leadership: The Conservative Promise.* [6]

At this writing, the incoming Trump administration has issued hundreds of Executive Orders, the unelected Elon Musk has rattled our economic and political cages, and the future of democracy is up for grabs in the U. S. [7-10]

References:

1.   Reich, R. Has the real meaning of America been lost? *San Francisco Chronicle*, February 20, 2018.

2.   Trump, DJ. Debate highlights sharp contrast in presentation. *New York Times*, June 29, 2024, A 12.

3.   Heritage Foundation's book, *Project 2025 Mandate for Leadership: The Conservative Promise,* April 2024.

4.   Johnston, David Cay. Apparently we are willing to give up our freedom, cowering to Trump . . . A power-mad con artist with no soul, February 11, 2025.

5.   Kahn, J. Critiquing Project 2025: Medicaid. *Health Justice Monitor*, June 29, 2024.

6.   Johnson, J. 'Gift to Corporate Greed': Dire warnings as Supreme Court scraps Chevron doctrine, *Common Dreams*, June 28, 2024.

Other Useful References.

7.   Applebaum, A. Democracy is losing the propaganda war. *The Atlantic* 353:5, June 2024, p. 40.

8.   Nader, R. In the public interest. What Donald Trump has revealed about our country. *The Progressive Populist,* February 15, 2025, p. 15.

9.   Legum, J. Update: the "deferred resignation" scam. *The Progressive Populist,* February 15, 2025, p. 15.

10.   Kuttner, R. The next financial crisis. *The Progressive Populist,* February 15, 2025, p. 12.

Chapter 11

Current Crisis In U. S. Health Care

Something inside the human spirit cries out against the injustice of inequality when you know people who have to choose between food and medicine in a country where CEOs make more in an hour than their lowest-paid employees make in a month.[1]

—The Reverend Dr. Barber II, WJ, president of the
North Carolina chapter of the NAACP, pastor at
Greenleaf Christian Church in Goldsboro, North
Carolina, and founder of Repairers of the Breach

The essence of medicine is so different from that of ordinary business that they are inherently at odds. Business concepts of good management may be useful in medical practice, but only to a degree. The fundamental ethos of medical practice contrasts sharply with that of ordinary commerce, and market principles do not apply to the relationship between physician and patient. Such insights have not stopped the growing domination of market ideology over medical professionalism.[2]

—Arnold S. Relman, M.D., nephrologist, editor of
The New England Journal of Medicine (1977 to 1991),
long-time advocate for physicians to retain an
ethical commitment to patients and safety.

In previous chapters we examined how Trumpcare has sabotaged the ACA and led to a far more dysfunctional health care system that increasingly fails the needs of ordinary Americans. It is now time to review the current crisis and chaos that cries out for fundamental reform. The goals of this chapter are (1) to briefly consider some societal trends that have allowed these changes to occur; and (2) to summarize the critical failings of Trumpcare today.

I.   *Historical Context*

Taking a step back, a strong case can be made that the uninterrupted progression of ever higher costs of private health insurance in the U. S. has brought the industry to its own crisis point. Earlier in this book, we have seen how costs have been consistently imposed by the industry. We have seen how total health care costs have increased to their present unaffordability.

Private insurers have accounted for these factors in their buildup to this point:

- upcoding, encouraged by insurers' profiteering;
- hospitals seeking higher reimbursements;
- increased spending on specialty drugs;
- government funding of privatized Medicare and Medicaid;
- corporate greed subsumes all of the above.

The corporate-controlled health care marketplace has left behind the traditional service ethic of the medical profession, as these markers reveal:

- Almost 70 percent of U. S. physicians now work for corporate   employers, especially hospital systems, under pressure to maximize revenues for their employers.
- Subversion of the electronic health record from its original goal to exchange medical and health care information to a billing instrument whereby physicians are pressured by their employers to up-code diagnoses for which care was not provided. [3]
- Private equity firms have been buying up hospitals, then cutting staff, reducing quality of care, loading them with debt, and finally selling them at a profit as many are forced to go into bankruptcy.[4]
- A similar approach has been taken for physician practices in primary care, emergency care, obstetrics-gynecology, mental health services, and other fields.[5]

- Investor-owned care consistently leads to higher costs and lower quality of care.[6]
- Private health insurerers have become skilled at manipulating medical loss ratios in order to avoid paying rebates to their insured. [7]
- The development of AI has raised questions about its value in clinical practice—can it be trusted to improve quality of care or not? [8]
- Based upon international data estimates, excess deaths attributable to the fragmented insurance system in the U. S. are likely to be over $190,000 per year.[9]
- The dissemination of medical information has become a growing industry of its own often rife with its own profiteering.[10]
- Price gouging by pharmaceutical companies still knows almost no bounds.[11]
- Employer-sponsored health insurance, previously the backbone of the health insurance industry, has become increasingly unaffordable for both employers and employees.
- Independent medical practices have all but disappeared while they have become burdened with more than 14 hours of work per week and surrounded with many managers.

II.   Crises Throughout the System: A Summary

Growing crises are rampant across all parts of U. S. health care despite a prevailing meme held by many conservatives that we have the best health care in the world. Policies on health care by the first Trump administration made health care worse, as these examples make clear.

1. Inadequate Access

Having adequate health insurance became more elusive under Trumpcare. There were 28 million Americans uninsured in 2018, with this number growing to 32 million in 2019 and 41 million in 2025, according to CBO estimates. Tens of millions will be underinsured, especially as the Trump administration promotes short-term plans of less than one year: with attractively low premiums but high deductibles and minimal coverage, hardly enough to be considered insurance. Most of these "cheap" short-term plans will exclude coverage of pre-existing conditions, preventive care, maternity care, mental health or substance abuse treatment.

With the ending of CSR payments, the insurance marketplace had become further destabilized. In response, insurers continued to raise premiums way beyond the cost of living for "inclusive plans." As two examples in Maryland, CareFirst BlueCross BlueShield requested a 91 percent increase on its PPO plans and Kaiser Permanente wanted a 37 percent hike on its HMO plans. Insurers were also exiting more markets, thereby increasingly segmenting risk pools to patients' disadvantage.

Trump's proposed rules for health insurance loosened insurance regulations, and called for expansion of association health plans. These proposals were widely opposed by consumer advocates, physician and nurse organizations, and trade groups representing insurers, hospitals, and clinics across the country.

When we look at specific parts of the system, the situation is dire, as these examples show.

- *Community health centers* are private, nonprofit organizations that provide primary care services to residents of a defined medically underserved area. They make up the largest primary care network for some 26 million people in underserved areas. A majority of their funding comes from the federal Community Health Center Fund, which has and continues to be on the chopping block by fiscal conservatives.
- *Women's health care.* The first Trump administration changed federal policy on women's reproductive health along ideologic lines that greatly restricted women's choices, all in the name of "pro-life." Even though the numbers of births and abortions were at an all-time low, Trump's proposed rules would forbid federally funded family planning clinics from referring women for abortions. They would also make

big changes in Title X, the family planning program that serves 4 million low-income people, including banning clinics from sharing physical space and financial resources with abortion providers. GOP efforts to defund Planned Parenthood continued, although 97 percent of its services are for preventive services such as contraceptive options, breast exams and screening for cervical cancer and sexually transmitted infections with only 3 percent for abortion services. Other regulatory proposals would emphasize "natural family planning" and abstinence.

- *Childrens' health care.* The Children's Health Insurance Program (CHIP) provided care for about 9 million children and 370,000 pregnant women nationwide. Trump's 2018 budget cut billions from CHIP over two years and limited eligibility for federal matching funds. Ongoing funding for this important program was in jeopardy and remained a political football between the states and the federal government. [12]
- *Mental health care.* Mental health disorders affect one in five adults in this country, and remain a leading cause of disability. But mental health care is poorly covered by private insurers, and payment for psychiatric services is so low that many health professionals avoided care of these patients. There is a critical shortage of state psychiatric beds across the country that force severely mentally ill patients to be held in emergency rooms, hospitals and jails while they waited for a bed, sometimes for weeks. [13]

2. Increasing disparities

Disparities are increasing for much of our population in our dysfunctional profit-oriented system, thereby placing a higher burden of illness, injury, disability and mortality experienced by one population group compared to another. These disparities could be based on such factors as race/ethnicity, socioeconomic status, age, location, gender and disability status. Disparities varied widely from one state to another.

Dr. H. Jack Geiger, founding member and past president of Physicians for Human Rights and past president of Physicians for Social Responsibility, says this about these persistent health disparities:

> *What we deal with in our work, quite apart from the extremes of genocide, is a variant of that: "Lives less worthy of life." When we say that the poor have a mortality rate that is multiple times the rate of the rich, when we say poor children die in our country and in the developing world at rates far higher than those of the better off, we are saying that we permit a condition which in effect says that they are less worthy of life. We are sending this message because we let it happen, because we have social policies that almost assure that it will happen, and we let it happen stubbornly and continually.*[14]

3. Unaffordable Costs of Care

The costs of health care in the U. S. continue to rise exponentially with no end in sight. A large and growing part of the population cannot afford necessary health care. The 2018 Milliman Medical Index reported that the typical working American family of four covered by an average employer-sponsored preferred provider organization (PPO) paid more than an average of $28,000 per year for health care, on insurance premiums, cost-sharing and forgone wage increases (for the employer contribution.) Those numbers in 2024 were $32,066 for a family of four for a year's health care. [15]

The median annual household income in the U. S. at that time was $59,358 and the Commonwealth Fund defined financial hardship for health care above 10 percent of annual income. These costs were almost one-half of annual income and clearly far beyond the wallets of ordinary Americans.

The Kaiser Family Foundation tracks these numbers in terms of the "medical bill score." Their polls have found that 31 percent of Americans ages 18 to 64 report that they or a family member face problems paying their health care bills; that number goes up to 57 percent if they are sick. As a result, 72 percent put off vacations or household purchases, 70 percent cut back on food, 59 percent used up all or most of their savings, and 41 percent took an extra job or worked more hours.[16]

Medical bills are a leading source of bankruptcy in the U. S. Even more commonly, medical debt exacts widespread damage to people's credit scores, with almost 40 percent of adults younger than 65 reporting lower credit scores for this reason.[17]

4. Inadequate Quality of Care

For those who think or assume that health care in this country is better than anywhere else, these sobering measures indicate the opposite:

- There has been a 50 percent increase in deaths from suicide, alcohol, and drug use since 2005.
- In 2016, average life expectancy at birth in the U. S. declined for a second year in a row.
- After trending downward for most of the last decade, rates of premature death from preventable or treatable causes were going up.
- 39 percent of adults in Mississippi and West Virginia are obese; one-quarter were obese even in states with the lowest rates.
- Across states, 41 percent to 66 percent of adults with symptoms of a mental illness (some of whom may not have been diagnosed) received no treatment in 2013-2015.
- Up to one-third of children needing mental health care in 2016 did not receive it, according to their parents.
- 29 percent of adults with employer-based insurance receive unneeded lower back imaging at diagnosis.
- Despite having Medicare, U. S. seniors with multiple chronic conditions or functional limitations report high rates of emergency department use and care coordination failures.[18]
- The two-thirds of the nation's nursing homes dependent on Medicaid funding have lower staffing and worse quality of care than others. [19]
- Missed visits and neglect were common for patients on hospice dying at home. [20]

We have a health care divide in this country which has much to do with where we live and one's ability to access high-quality health care and live a healthy life. Figure 11.1 shows these stark differences between better-than-average states and worse-than-average states. Figure 11.2 displays the extent to which mortality in this country's health care system falls behind fifteen other countries in mortality.

5. *Instability and Volatility*

Our incoherent health care non-system has never been more unstable as the roles of insurers, hospitals, clinics, and corporate stakeholders continue to change, mostly chasing larger market share and higher revenues. Here are just three examples of the changing health care landscape without much clarity for its future.

- UnitedHealth, one of the largest private insurers, purchased DeVita, a large for-profit chain of dialysis centers with almost 300 clinics [21]; before this purchase, UnitedHealth was already working with more than 30,000 physicians across 230 urgent care clinics and 200 surgery centers.
- CVS Health, the second largest drugstore chain, bought Aetna, the third largest insurer; this could lead to a network of clinics in almost 10,000 drugstores around the country.[21]
- Dignity Health and Catholic Health Initiatives planned to become a national chain of Catholic hospitals and clinics in 28 states with 139 hospitals and more than 25,000 physicians and other clinicians. [22]

Through these mergers, corporate stakeholders were trying to expand into new roles within a turbulent transformation of health care. No longer would physicians' offices be the hub of the system as urgent care centers and retail clinics proliferate in new locations, including drug stores and shopping malls. A battle was raging among competing interests for control of the primary care patient, which will determine where patients are hospitalized, where they fill their prescriptions, and where they receive laboratory tests and imaging procedures.

Patients were left out of this increasingly volatile system, with merging corporate stakeholders pursuing their own self-interest in a less accountable system rather than service to patients.

Figure 11.1

AMERICA'S HEALTH CARE DIVIDE
STATE HEALTH SYSTEM PERFORMANCE
VARIES ACROSS THE COUNTRY

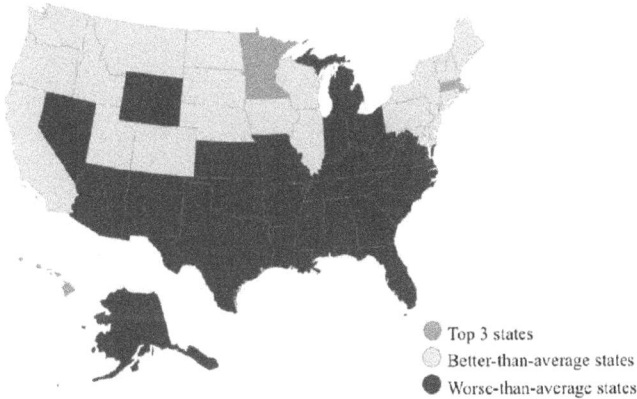

● Top 3 states
◐ Better-than-average states
● Worse-than-average states

Source: 2018 Scorecard on State Health System Performance.
The Commonwealth Fund

Figure 11.2

OVERALL STATE HEALTH SYSTEM PERFORMANCE:
U.S. LAGS OTHER COUNTRIES:
MORTALITY AMENABLE TO HEALTH CARE

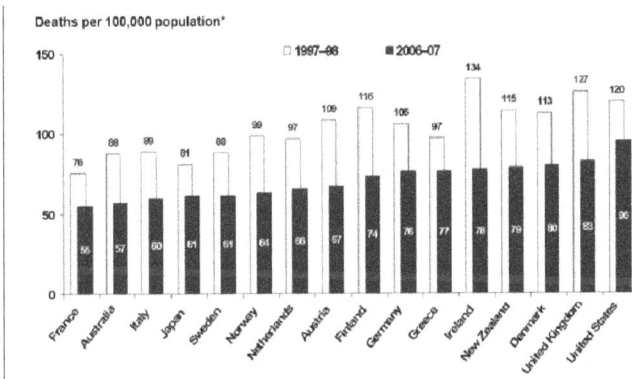

Source: *Mirror, Mirror, A Portrait of the Failing U.S. Health System,*
The Commonwealth Fund.

Patients will likely see less choice of health care providers, higher costs, more fragmentation and less continuity of care. Meanwhile, they face churning of insurance coverage, which will become even worse if the GOP succeeds in cuts to Medicare and Medicaid. Some insurers are now even questioning the need for emergency room visits, thereby imposing large uncovered costs on patients for the follow-up care that results.

6. *Deteriorating Safety Net*

Within all this turbulence in health care, the nation's safety net under the Trump administration is falling apart. These examples show how vulnerable lower-income Americans now struggle to survive in an increasingly cruel and uncaring society.

- 41 million Americans, larger than the combined populations of Texas, Michigan, and Maine, are classified by the U. S. Department of Agriculture as "food insecure." Family food insecurity exceeds 14 percent of those living in urban and rural areas.[23] The Supplemental Nutrition Assistance Program (SNAP), commonly known as food stamps, is threatened by the loss of 18 billion in 2026, the loss of 193,000 jobs and loss of state and local tax revenues by $1.8 billion. [24] Food stamps also fail to cover the actual costs of a low-income meal in 99 percent of U. S. counties and the District of Columbia.[25]

- Subject to congressional approval, Trump wanted to rescind $5 billion for the popular Children's Health Insurance Program (CHIP). After signing the March 2018 spending bill, the president was pushed by conservatives in Congress to cut the federal deficit, which was projected to be almost $1 trillion in 2019.[26]

- Women are more likely than men to have low incomes and be the primary caretakers of their children. Since 40 million women are on Medicaid, they are especially vulnerable to cuts in safety net programs. Despite these facts, the first Trump administration was disinvesting in women and families by such means as cuts in food stamps, reducing family planning funding, promoting short-term insurance policies without maternity coverage, imposing new work requirements for Medicaid, and proposals that would raise rents for low-income families.[27]

- About 7 million retirees who have depended on long-term care insurance are facing steep premium increases for less coverage. More than one-half of U. S. adults are expected to need nursing home or other care services. Long-term care typically costs at least $100,000 a year per individual. The long-term care insurance industry, however, is dying, with most insurers leaving this market.[28]
- Medicaid coverage, unstable at best and facing likely cutbacks at both federal and state levels, varies greatly from one state to another.[29] Nursing homes and group homes in Louisiana give us one current example of what these cuts can mean in one state. If proposed cuts are made, more than 30,000 Medicaid recipients will lose their benefits and face eviction.
- The 2nd Trump administration has just increased funding for higher payouts to private health insurers of Medicare Advantage. [31]

Katrina vanden Heuvel, editor and publisher of *The Nation*, comments on this dire situation:

> *The administration is using the pretense of fiscal responsibility to slash programs for the poor and people of color . . . When you have policies that take away the human rights of the poor and make women and children prey, then you have a nation that can't survive.* [32]

The ugly underbelly of conservatives' attacks on welfare is exposed and fueled by Trump's racist rhetoric and the white supremacy movement to Make America Great Again. A recent study by two sociology researchers at the University of California Berkeley and Stanford University concluded that opposition to welfare has risen sharply among whites. Racial anxiety appeared to be driving their calls for deeper cuts in welfare programs. [33]

Concluding comment

As a result of all this turmoil within health care, we have a rudderless, unaccountable "system" without a moral compass, aided and abetted by an enabling hands-off government. Patients and families are losing out as corporate giants vie for a bigger piece of the health care pie. Taxpayers can't afford this wasteful system at either the state or federal level.

The Senate approved the choice of Robert F. Kennedy, Jr., as the new head of the Department of Health and Human Services. A vaccine denier, it was controversial on that count, especially with a growing national measles outbreak for which he wants to counter with cod liver oil. In addition, he has refused to divest millions of dollars that could result from pending anti-vaccine lawsuits, an indication that departmental fraud may well be extended by this choice. [34]

Another potentially important recent development was a $2.8 billion dollar payout promising reforms the Blue Cross Blue Shield Association and other health insurers focused on, during the process involving pre-authorization of services and related matters.[35]

This could improve and update needed discussions about processes involving more than one-third of all Americans and U. S. medical providers.

In today's polarized political climate, we have just two major options—continue with Trumpcare as the sabotaged version of the ACA or support real reform through a single-payer Medicare for All national system committed to the common good of all Americans.

As we face health care reform today, delayed for these many decades, we can take heart from these words from Ralph Nader's recently published book, *Civil Self-respect*:

. . .we must acquire knowledge within the context of justice and connect what we know to civic action. [36]

—Nader, R., *Civic Self-Respect*, 2025

References:

1. Barber II, WJ. The Third Reconstruction: How a Moral Movement Is Overcoming the Politics of Division and Fear. Boston. *Beacon Press*, 2016, p. xiii.
2. Relman, AS. Medical professionalism in a commercialized health care market. *JAMA* 298 (22): 2669, 2007.
3. Geyman, JP. Private equity looting of U. S. health care: An under- recognized and uncontrolled scourge. *Int. J Health Services* on line, November 3, 2022.
4. Abelson, R, Sanger-Katz, M, "The cash machine was insatiable": How
5. Zucker, H. Where have all the doctors gone? AARP.Org/Bulletin, January/February 2025, p. 10.
6. Bhatia, A. Changes in patient care experience after private equity acquisition of U. S. hospitals. *JAMA*, January 9, 2025.
7. Potter, W. WSJ: How United Health's diagnosis game rakes in billions from Medicare. healthcareuncovered@substack.com>, January 7, 2025.
8. Wartman, SA, Densen, P. Will artificial intelligence undermine the practice of medicine? *The Pharos*, Autumn, 2024, p. 4.
9. Kahn, J. Deaths due to willful systemic failings are violent, too. Health Justice Monitor, December 10, 2024.
10. Potter, W. healthcareuncovered.@substack.com, 2025.
11. Potter, W. Big insurance 2022: Revenues reached $1.25 trillions thanks to sucking billions out of the pharmacy supply chain—and taxpayers' pockets. *Wendell Potter's Health Care uncovered*, February 27, 2023.
12. Itkowitz, D, Somashekhar, S. States prepare to shut down children's health programs if Congress doesn't act. *The Washington Post*, November 23, 2017.
13. Davis, K. Single-payer system is the solution for mental health care, panelists say. *American Journal of Managed Care*, May 7, 2018.
14. Geiger, HJ. Why we do what we do, speech. Doctors for Global Health, August 2002.
15. Milliman Medical Index, May 2024, for family of four—$32,066.
16. Luthra, S. When credit scores become casualties of health care. *Kaiser Health News,* May 9, 2018
17. Radley, DC, McCarthy, D, Hayes, SL. 2018 Scorecard on State Health System Performance. New York. *The Commonwealth Fund.*
18. Osborn, R, Doty, MM, Moulds, D et al. Older Americans were sicker and faced more financial barriers to health care than counterparts in other countries. *Health Affairs*, November 15, 2017.
19. Rau, J. Why glaring quality gaps among nursing homes are likely to grow if Medicaid is cut. *Kaiser Health News,* September 28, 2017.
20. Aleccia, J, Bailey, M, de Marco, H. No one is coming. Hospice patients abandoned at death's door. *Kaiser Health News*, October 26, 2017.
21. Abelson, R. United Health buys large doctors group as lines blur in health

care. *New York Times*, December 6, 2017.

22. Tracer, Z. Forget Amazon. Health companies really want to be United Health. *Bloomberg News*, December 4, 2017.

23. de la Merced, MJ, Abelson, R. CVS to buy Aetna for $69 billion in a deal that may reshape the health industry. *New York Times*, December 3, 2017.

24. Alterman, E. Hungry and invisible. *The Nation*, November 13, 2017.

25. Rampal, C., Congress takes food from 2 million poor people-and dosen't even save money, *The Washington Post*, May 17, 2018

26. Waxman, E. How far do SNAP benefits fall short of covering the cost of a meal? *Urban Institute*, February 22, 2018.

27. Galewitz, P. 4 takeaways from Trump's plan to rescind CHIP funding. *Kaiser Health News*, May 8, 2018.

28. Bernstein, J, Katch, H. Cutting support for economically vulnerable women is no way to celebrate Mother's Day. *The Washington Post*, May 11, 2018.

29. Scism, L. Safety net frays for millions of retirees. *Wall Street Journal*, January 17, 2018: A1.

30. Galewitz, P. 4 takeaways from Trump's plan to rescind CHIP funding. *Kaiser Health News*, May 8, 2018.

31. Mathews, K.W. Private manager plans to get a big boost. *Wall Street Journal*, April 8, 2025

32. vanden Heuvel, K. Trump's brutal policies target the most vulnerable Americans, *The Progressive Populist*, June 15, 2018, p. 12.

33. Dewey, C. White America's racial resentment is the real impetus to welfare cuts, study says. *The Washington Post*, May 30, 2018.

34. <robertreich@substack.com. January 28, 2025.>

35. Potter, W. *Changing the Blues: Inside the largest antitrust settlement in U. S. health care. January 28, 2025.*

36. Nader, R., *Civic Self-respect, Seven Stories Press*, New York, N.Y., 2025 p.138.

Chapter 12

Long Overdue For The U.S.: National Health Insurance

The federal government should not play a huge role in health care regulation. The only way the government should be involved, they have to make sure those companies are financially strong, so that if they have a catastrophic event or they have a miscalculation, they have plenty of money. Other than that, it's private.

—Donald Trump, as presidential candidate, in talk to *The Hill* [1]

Dana Milbank, political columnist for *The Washington Post*, brings us this forecast of Trump's second term:

We're already back to the chaos, caprice and over-reach. Any hope that he might moderate—in truth, this was never more than a fantasy—has already been dashed . . . His administration is going to be just as incompetent as it was last time- maybe more so. . . The man is too unstable to be competent. [2]

The Trump quote is typical of many by Donald Trump in that it reveals so little understanding of the problems and dynamics of our health care system. It fits with his philosophy and that of congressional Republicans favoring deregulation and a limited role of the federal government in health care. The Millbank quote represents what we may come to expect as the second example of Trumpcare takes shape.

This chapter has three goals: (1) to describe changes to the Affordable Care Act that were made by the first Trump administration under a supposed "value-based" initiative free market approach; (2) to show who wins vs. loses under a public national health insurance as a future reformed health care system; and (3) to briefly comment on 2025 geopolitics of health care as we build political support for national health insurance.

I. *Alternatives for Health Care*

Four different approaches to health care are compared in Table 12.1 and Table 12.2. In his first term Trump supported the "free market" approaches to health care: (1) Continuation of the Affordable Care Act. (2) Public Option. (3) Medicare Advantage with profitability to private corporate interests and (4) Medicare for All, a nonprofit National Health Insurance.

Looking ahead to Trump's second term, Timothy Noah, staff writer at *The New Republic*, observed:

> *Trump wants to cut taxes and halt regulations: beyond that, his policies are entirely transactional. He'll do something if it helps him or enriches him or gratifies his bottomless need to be cheered at political rallies. He'll avoid anything that doesn't do those things.*[3]

Table 12.1 is a comparison of nine VALUES among four health care options. The first three options serve the values of the few, the private corporate stakeholders and their stakeholders, while the fourth option, Medicare for All, serves the common good and is the only option that supports all nine positive values.

Table 12.2 is a comparison of eight positive EVIDENCE criteria. The first three do not meet any of the criteria and only the fourth option, Medicare for All, meets all of the criteria.

It is clear that only Medicare for All - National Health Insurance is the only alternative which meets all of the values and evidence criteria which are essential for effective health insurance for all U.S. residents. It will provide reform for our current out-of-control corporatized mega-merged "system" and is committed to the common good.

TABLE 12.1
Value-Based Comparison of Four Alternatives

	ACA	PUBLIC OPTION	MEDICARE ADVANTAGE FOR ALL	MEDICARE FOR ALL
Health care a human right	No	No	No	Yes
Commodity for sale?	Yes	Yes	Yes	No
Profit vs. service ethic	Profit	Profit	Profit	Service
Full choice of physician & hospital	No	No	No	Yes
Accessable, reliable, efficient?	No	No	No	Yes
Not for profit, reduced waste?	No	No	No	Yes
Population-based, shared risk?	No	No	No	Yes
Science-based?	No	No	No	Yes
Common good, public interest?	No	No	No	Yes

Sources: Geyman, J. P., *Value and Evidence Based Comparison of Four Reform Alternatives, The Future of of U.S. Health Care?: Corporate Power versus the Common Good, NOVA Science Publishers*, 2022, p.140.

TABLE 12.2
Evidence-Based Comparison of Four Alternatives

	ACA	PUBLIC OPTION	MEDICARE ADVANTAGE FOR ALL	MEDICARE FOR ALL
Access	Restricted	Restricted	Restricted	Unrestricted
Choice	Restricted	Restricted	Restricted	Unrestricted
Cost containment	Never	Never	Never	Yes
Quality of care	Unacceptable	Unacceptable	Unacceptable	Improved
Bureaucracy	Large, wasteful	Large, wasteful	Large, wasteful	Much reduced
Universal coverage	Never	Never	Never	Yes
Accountability	No	No	No	Yes
Sustainability	No	No	No	Yes

April 2025 planning by the Trump administration:

We can expect a battle royal between the private health insurance industry hoping to extend its privateering ways through privatized Medicare Advantage. Already in April 2025, the Committee For a Responsible Federal Budget has brought forward a plan for overpayment of Medicare Advantage by a staggering $1.2 trillion over the coming decade while continuing favorable risk selection through upcoding. [4]

This experienced leader of the reform movement since the late 1980s brought this fresh view of what has transpired over the years:

> We need to envision a health system where the distribution of infrastructure and resources is not left to the dictates of the market but rationally planned according to the needs of communities—and the certainty of future disasters. It requires discarding the false promise of anarchical medical competition as the salve of our healthcare cost crisis.[5]

> —Gaffney, A. Past President of Physicians for a National Health Program and author of *To Heal Humankind: The Right to Health in History*

II. Winners and Losers: Trumpcare vs. National Health Insurance

With Trump now in his second term Presidency, we can count on unaffordable costs and prices of care, poor access and quality of care in the same way as in past years. As health care expert Dr. Don McCanne observed after the shooting death of Brian Thomson, UnitedHealth's CEO:

> More than ever, for the health of our nation, we see that it is imperative that we eliminate this industry and replace it with a single payer system, a carefully improved version of Medicare that serves all of us while making it equitable, comprehensive, accessible, and affordable.[6]

> —Don McCanne, M.D., Past President of Physicians for a National Health Program

Other leaders agree that violence has no place in our opposition to what private health insurers have brought the nation. Bernie Sanders, Independent senator from Vermont, added:

The current system is broken, it is dysfunctional, it is cruel, and it is wildly inefficient—far too expensive. The reason we have not joined virtually every other major country on Earth in guaranteeing healthcare to all people as a human right is the political power and financial power of the insurance industry and drug companies.[7]

As we should have learned many years ago, it is finally time for the U. S. to learn and avoid the downsides of profit-based employer health insurance.

U. S. National Health Insurance

Winners

1. **Patients of all ages.** Regardless of their health conditions, they will be immediately covered with full access to all necessary care, with full choice of provider and hospital, and with no cost sharing at the point of care. Women will gain by having full access to all reproductive health services, thereby gaining control over their own bodies and family choices without political barriers. Each individual will have an NHI card to make an appointment with a physician or medical care provider.

2. **Medical need, not ability to pay** is the basis of NHI.

3. **Quality and outcome of care.** As all U.S. residents gain access to all necessary health care, the quality and outcomes of their care will improve. That is especially true for those population subgroups that have inadequate access under the present system.

4. **Equity across the health care system.** National health insurance will bring equity across the system, provide solid funding of safety net programs in the country and eliminate today's health care divide from one state to another. NHI will build on the reliable performance demonstrated by traditional, non-privatized Medicare for more than 50 years. Rural areas will be better served with NHI as hubs of accessible care to residents of large areas.

5. **Physicians and other health professionals.** They will join the winners' circle for NHI with administrative simplification and gaining more time for patient care. They will experience higher practice satisfaction, less burnout, and have more autonomy in clinical decision-making. It will be a welcome change to no longer have to deal with the current enormous bureaucracy of pre-authorizations for care and responding to the many restrictions imposed by different private insurers.

6. **Hospitals.** With many millions of patients now underinsured or uninsured, the hospital industry today is under fire by market forces that compel hundreds of hospitals to shrink, reinvent themselves, or even close. With national health insurance, the need to keep hospitals open will be based on annual budget negotiations.

7. **Employers.** They are increasingly frustrated and burdened by the rising costs of providing employer-sponsored health insurance to their employees. Employers will be relieved of their role in providing health insurance. They will gain a healthier workforce at less cost, thereby becoming more competitive in a global economy.

8. **Mental Health.** Longstanding gaps in coverage of mental health care will be a thing of the past.

9. **Public Health.** This essential area of service to the public on national health issues will receive more funding.

10. **Taxpayers.** Progressive taxation, with elimination of today's waste and profiteering of the private multi-payer financing system, will be a great advance in a new culture of care. It will be affordable for everyone because of sharing risk across all 338 million of us in an efficient, not-for-profit financing system.

Losers

1. **Private Health Insurers.** They have had their chance for many decades and have failed the common good. The large labyrinth of corporate middlemen profiteering through-out the medical-industrial complex fails the public interest. Privatized Medicare and Medicaid have shown to have higher costs, because of profits, than the publicly administered programs. Government reports estimate that

Medicare Advantage plans may be overpaid by at least $43 Billion per year. [8]

2.   **Corporate stakeholders.** Ranging from pharmaceutical companies to medical device manufacturers, they will not compete as in the past. However, they will have the opportunity to compete based on the quality and efficacy of their products in one big market through bulk purchasing.

Transition:

Implementing a new national health insurance program will take time. For example, all the benefits of the current Medicare for All Act, which has been introduced in Congress, would go into effect two years after the date of its enactment.

Critics of single-payer NHI say that it will be too disruptive. History tells us the opposite. When Medicare and Medicaid were enacted in 1965, even in a time of 3x5 cards and other paper records, the change was almost seamless for patients, and care began right away. Disruption will occur, however, in the private administrative sector, but that is needed to rectify its many problems that have been sold to us under the false banner of "more efficiency in the private sector." (Table 12.3)

Table 12.3

WINNERS AND LOSERS UNDER NATIONAL HEALTH INSURANCE

Winners	Losers
All U.S. residents	Private health insurers
Physicians, other health professionals	Corporate middlemen
	Corporate stakeholders
Hospitals	Privatized Medicare
Employers	Privatized Medicaid
Mental health care	Displaced workers
Public health	Lobbyists
Federal and state governments	
Taxpayers	

Source: Geyman, J. P., *Common Sense, U.S. Health Care At A Crossroads, Is it finally time for National Health Insurance, Copernicus Healthcare*, p.12, 2025

III. Health Care Politics in Turmoil

We can expect that chaos will reign in Trump's second attempt to administer U. S. health care. The GOP and the Trump team, as members of the billionaire class, have taken on a controlling role, which reminds us of the late 1920s, which led to the most transformative time in the 1930s as the country changed course in support ot the common good for most Americans.

Today, however, we have an oligarchy, siphoning off the wealth of the U. S. in support of a conflicted felon President as they support tax cuts for the wealthy. [9] As Jim Hightower has pointed out:

> *Trump and Musk aren't reforming our government, they're sabotaging it... Soft words like "efficiency" are their knives for castrating government of, by, and for, The People, allowing a cabal of Trump and Musk, and allied financial elites to impose a moneyed monarchy over America. But remember our history—we democratic rebels won all-out wars in the 1770s and 1860s to defeat them. So toughen-up here they come again.* [10]

In the hands-off, deregulated approach taken by the Trump administration to health care, corporate interests thrive and they have been able to game the system. Dr. Mehmet Oz leads the Centers for Medicare and Medicaid Services, which administers privatized Medicare Advantage for All. In that capacity, he can overpay government money for that program by a staggering $1.2 trillion over the next decade. Together with upcoding, those over-payments will drive-up profits for private health insurers in undetected ways. [11]

IV. The Way Forward

In order to evaluate and come to grips as a society with which of these two alternatives to pursue—Trumpcare or National Health Insurance (single-payer Medicare for All) We must first answer a fundamental question: who is the health care system for? Is it for patients and families or for corporate interests? If the GOP is to hold to its claimed conservative principles, Republicans should be able to review this book and join Democrats to formulate an answer to this question in the public interest.

Our task is to build political support in the country for National Health Insurance. Following is a beginning:

- *Urge the Democratic party* to include national health insurance on their platform.
- Support Congressional leaders and their committees
  1. Pramila Jayapal has just reintroduced the Medicare for All Act in the 2025-26 House of Representatives: H.R. 3421
  2. Bernie Sanders introduced the Medicare for All Act in the 2023-24 Senate: S.A. 1655
- Contact organizations that support National Health Insurance.
  1. American Nurses Association
  2. BOLD! Democrats
  3. HealthCare-NOW!
  4. Indivisible
  5. National Nurses United
  6. NextGen America
  7. Physicians for a National Health Program
  8. Progressive Democrats of America
  9. Public Citizen
  10. The Lincoln Project

Ruth Ben-Ghiat, expects that Musk's Department of Government Efficiency (DOGE) will be "an Orwellian test case for disrupting society through economic "shock events" that paralyze governance and create mass misery." [12] As an expert on autocracies around the world and author of the 2020 book *Strongmen: Mussolini to the Present*, she brings this advice from her own manifesto, *Lucid*, to carry us forward with hope and perseverance:

> *Lucid is a space of caring and solidarity where we help each other process the losses we suffer due to negligent and repressive governance, racism, misogyny, homophobia, environmental plunder, and gun violence. We need open hearts and transparent communications to recover and rebuild trust, including trust in our collective power to stand up to situations that threaten our dignity and freedoms.* [13]

References:

1. Donald Trump, as presidential candidate, in talk to *The Hill*
2. Millbank, Dana, *The Washington Post*
3. Noah, Timothy, *The New Republic*
4. Potter, W., Rettino, J. J. Congress to GAO: Follow the Medicare Advantage Money,,<*healthcare uncovered,substack*>, April 22, 2025.
5. Gaffney, A., Past President of Physicians for a National Health Program, *P.N.H.P.*
6. Don McCanne, M.D., Would single payer be good for America? *P.N.H.P.*, https:// pnhp.org/publications/would_single_payer_be_good_for_america.php
7. Corbett, J., Sanders Says 'Political Movement,' Not Murder, Is the Path to Medicare for All, *Common Dreams*, Dec 12, 2024
8. Potter, W., CMS's "significant expansion" of audits has made UnitedHealth's bad year even worse. <healthcareuncovered@substack.com> June 3, 2025
9. Jones, S, Easley, J. Politics will be defined by class not party over the next four years. *Daily Politics USA*, December 12, 2024.
10. Hightower, J. Trump and Musk aren't reforming our government, they are sabotaging it. <*jimhightower@substack.com*> April 15, 2025.
11. Ibid #4
12. Ben-Ghiat, R.A new kind of coup: Trump and Musk are updating the autocratic playbook
13. Ben-Ghiat, R. Elon Musk: a new and sinister force in government. <*lucid@substack.com*>.

INDEX

Note: Figures are indicated by (f) and tables by (t) following the page number.

A

Abortion rights
    seven states affirming, 84
    states where abortion is legal, banned or under threat (map), 86f
    Supreme Court striking down Roe v. Wade (2022), 83
Adams, John, 107
Affordable Care Act of 2010 (ACA)
    administrative bureaucracy, 91–92
    conflicting interests and goals, 32
    corporate alliance for health care reform, 32, 33t
    corruption by outside money, 31–34
    insurers gaming system for higher profits, 19
    limitations of, 69, 118–119
    minimal federal oversight, 102
    passage and continuing opposition to, 3–4
    private interests prioritized over quality health care, 16–17
    sabotage by Republicans, 4
    unaffordable premiums, 64
    value-based initiatives for patient care, 107–108
Affordable health care
    annual and lifetime limits by insurers, 76
    barriers to, 70–77
    declining access to, 69–80
    government involvement and, 119–120
    health costs and, 71
    high cost sharing, adverse effects, 73–74
    inequality and declining access to, 79
    out-of-pocket costs limiting affordability for seniors, 74
    problems paying medical bills, 76–77
    restrictive Medicaid changes, 75

total health care spending, 77–79

Trumpcare worsening access to, 119–120

unaffordable health insurance limiting access, 71–73

uninsured population and, 70–71

American Medical Association (AMA), 2

Angell, Marcia, 69, 119

Ansell, David, 79

Applebaum, Anne, 123

Assisted living facilities, 117

Association health plans, expansion of, 128

Auble, Daniel, 28

Azar, Alex, 29, 30

B

Baker, Dean, 36, 61

Barber II, W.J., 125

Ben-Ghiat, Ruth, 148

Bertolini, Mark, 20

Biden, Joe, on oligarchy of the ultra-wealthy, 36

Biden administration

FDA regulatory oversight, 107

major legislation under, 34–36

Biennial Health Insurance Survey (2024), 66–67

Billing activities, costs for primary care physicians, 94

Biotechnology Innovation Organization, 27

Blumenthal, Richard, 105

Bolt, Chad, 63

Boushey, Heather, 79

Brown, Sherwood, 9

C

Cassidy, Bill, 61

Center for Reproductive Rights, 85

Centers for Medicare and Medicaid (CMS), 4

Chen, Hui, 95

Cherry picking of patients by insurers, 55

Children's Health Insurance Program (CHIP), 129, 134

Chittister, Joan D., 86–87

Chomsky, Noam, 22–23

Churchill, Winston, 91

Clinton Health Plan (CHP), 3

CMS, 4

Cohen, D. and Mikaelien, A., The Privatization of Everything: How the Plunder of Public Goods Transformed America and How We Can Fight Back, 43

Common good, 123

Community health centers, as primary care networks, 128

Comstock Act, 85

Consumer driven health care, 13

Corcoran, Michael, 80

Corlette, Sabrina, 61

Corporate greed and privateering
    conflicts of interest between industry and government, 28–29
    disruption of U.S. health care and, 27–37
    General Motors and, 8
    PhRMA as poster child for, 27–31

Corporations
    CEO compensation vs. middle-income wealth, 5, 6f
    for-profit health care and ownership of facilities, 13–14
    as losers under national health insurance, 145
    marketing of health care, 14

Cost-sharing, health care utilization and, 73–74

Cost-sharing reduction (CSR)
    Affordable Care Act and, 19
    ending of payments and destabilization of insurance payments, 128
    insurance premium increases and, 20, 62

COVID-19 vaccines, price gouging by manufacturers, 30

D

Deaths, U.S., attributable to fragmented insurance system, 127

Democracy in America? What Has Gone Wrong and What We Can Do About It (Page and Gilens), 34

Department of Goverment Efficiency, 108

Deregulation of health care, 101–105
    as deconstruction of administrative state, 101
    drug industry, 103–104

first Trump administration, 107

hospices, 105

hospital industry, 102–103

insurance industry, 101–102

laboratory tests, 105

medical device industry, 104

nursing homes, 104–105

regulation in the public interest, 106–109

surgery centers, 103

Drug Enforcement Agency (DEA), 114–115

Drug industry. See Pharmaceutical industry

E

Early retirees, and affordable health care barriers, 71

Economy, U.S., and health care industry, 15

Elderly persons

loss of ACA protections, 63

out-of-pocket costs limiting health care affordability, 74

Electronic health records

fraud enabled by, 96

up-coding of diagnoses, 126

Emergency medical services (EMS), privatization of, 53

Employers, as winners under national health insurance, 144

Employer-sponsored insurance, 66

Ensuring Patient Access and Effective Drug Enforcement Act of 2016, 114–115

Environmental Protection Agency (EPA), dismantling of, 118

Equity across health care system, national health insurance and, 143–144

F

Field, Robert, 17

Fischer, Will, 51

Food and Drug Administration (FDA), 107, 113–114

Food insecurity, 134

Food stamps, 134

Fraud

single-payer financing as solution for, 99

in U.S. health care billing, 96–99

Free market, and health care reform, 12

Freedom Caucus, opposition to ACA, 3–4
Freedom of Access to Clinic Entrances Act, 85
Frum, David, 22

G

Gaffney, A., 142
Geiger, H. Jack, 130
General Motors, corporate greed of, 8
Gilbert, Lisa, 9
Gingrich, Newt, 44
Goozner, Merrill, 48
Graffney, Adam, 47, 142
Gross domestic product (GDP), post-pandemic recovery, 35f

H

Hacker, Jacob, 21–22
Hartmann, Thom, 39
Hayek, Friedrich A., 11
Health care, U.S. See also Privatization of health care
 administrative costs, 92
 alternatives for, 140–141, 141t
 beneficiaries of system, 147
 as commodity, 15, 106
 corporate mergers, 132
 corporate privateering and disruption of, 27–37
 corporations and myth of efficiency, 12
 current crisis in, 125–136
 deregulation of, 101–105
 deteriorating accountability under Trump administration, 113–118
 economic impact, 15
 ending of CSR payments and destabilization of insurance marketplace, 128
 fraud in, 96–99
 "free market" approaches, 140
 goals for health care systems (Light), 112–113
 health care divide by state, 132, 133f
 inadequate access, 128–129
 inadequate oversight and accountability, 111–121
 increased government involvement required for improving, 120

increasing bureaucracy in, 91–93

increasing disparities, 129–130

instability and volatility of, 132–134

Medicaid expenditures (1966-2015), 72–73, 72f

medical bills as leading cause of bankruptcy, 131

mortality amenable to health care, U.S. vs. other countries, 133f

multi-payer vs. single-payer accountability for health care, 112–113

political bribery through corporate lobbying, 106, 106f

political turmoil in, 146–147

quality of care, inadequacies of, 131–132

regulation in the public interest, 106–109

as social good, 69

traditional Medicare vs. Medicare Advantage costs, 93

unaffordability of, 130–131

Health care accountability

deterioration under Trump administration, 113–118

government role in ensuring, 118–120

Health care industries

for-profit, cost containment not possible under, 17–18

lobbying targeting both political parties, 34

Health care marketplace

corporate-controlled, abandoning service ethic of medical profession, 126–127

inefficiencies of privatization, 53

Health care reform

barriers to, 11–24

Clinton Health Plan (CHP), 3

corporate alliance under ACA, 32, 33t

evidence-based comparison of alternatives, 141, 141t

failed attempts, 16–22

failure and loss of democratic process, 22

financing system reform and, 18

for-profit business ethic reform required in deregulated market, 17–18

insurance and overuse of health care services as myth, 13

large risk pool size required for efficient health insurance coverage, 19

larger government role needed for, 21–22

myths and memes affecting, 12–13

private sector efficiency as myth, 12

reform attempts, 1–10

value-based comparison of alternatives, 140–141, 141t

Health insurance

deaths attributable to fragmented system in U.S., 127

health care impact of high deductibles, 13

manipulation of medical loss ratios, 127

multi-payor, payment abuses, 116

short-term plans proposed by Trump administration, 115

unaffordability of private insurance as crisis, 126

Health insurance, employer-based

as barrier to reform, 91

increasing unaffordability of, 127

Health insurance industry

administrative costs, 93–94

government friendliness toward, 19

health care impact of high deductibles, 13

increase in insurers since 1980s, 4

Medicare and Medicaid supporting, 5f

multipayor, as barrier to universal coverage, 19–20

overuse of health services as myth, 13

private insurers as losers under national health insurance, 144–145

prohibitive cost of health insurance, 20–21

Health maintenance organizations (HMOs)

administrative bureaucracy of, 91–92

private Medicare overpayments to, 44

Health professionals, as winners under national health insurance, 144

Health safety net

deterioration of, 65, 134–136

women's vulnerability to cuts in, 134–135

Herbert, Bob, 16–17

Heuvel, Katrina vanden, 135

Hijacked: The Road to Single Payer in the Aftermath of Stolen Health Care Reform (Geyman), 16

Hospices
    fraud and abuse in, 98, 105
Hospital industry
    mergers and market-power price increases, 32
    overregulation of, 102
    price gouging, 30
    as winners under national health insurance, 144

I

Icahn, Carl, 118
In vitro services, and fetal personhood, 85
Independent medical practices, disappearance of, 127
Insulin, and price gouging by manufacturers, 30
Insurance industry, deregulation of, 101–102
International Health Policy Survey of Older Adults (Commonwealth Fund,
    2017), 54

J

Johnston, David Cay, 123
Joint Commission on Accreditation of Hospitals, 102

K

Kahn, Jim, 78
Kaiser Family Foundation, medical bill scores, 130–131
Kennedy, Robert F., Jr., 86, 136
Khan, Lisa, 36, 107
Kimmel, Jimmy, 61
Klobuchar, Amy, 105

L

Laboratory tests, 105
Lawrence, Hal, 86
Leggitt, Larry, 96
Lemon dropping of patients by insurers, 55
Light, Donald, 112–113
Lobbying industry, 34
Long-term care insurance, 134
Lucia, Kevin, 62

M

Marino, Tom, 114

McCanne, Don, 108, 142

Medicaid, 116

    impacts of non-expansion in 2022, 64

    instability of coverage, 135

    Personal Care Services, fraud and abuse in, 98

    privatization, negative impacts, 48, 98

    program cuts affecting women, 135

    restrictive changes to, 75

    revenue growth and privatization, 30

    states banning abortion opposing expansion, 64, 65f

    tightening of eligibility requirements, 63

    work requirements, 63, 75

Medical device industry, 104

Medical identity theft, 98

Medical information, dissemination of, 127

Medical loss ratios, manipulation of, 127

Medical need, national health insurance and, 143

Medical-industrial complex, 14–15

Medicare

    dangers of privatization, 116

    fee-for-service criteria, 54

    lost patient protections affecting, 63

    overpayments to private plans, 46–47

    political assumptions shaping current structure, 48–49

    private plans discriminating against sicker enrollees, 48

    privatization of, 46–49

    privatized vs. public, comparative features, 47t

    as social insurance, 54

Medicare Advantage

    fraudulent billing practices, 98

    overpayments to companies, 46

    privatization and revenue growth, 30, 32

Medicare-for-All. See National health insurance (NHI)

Medication abortion, 85

Mental health care
    inadequacy of services for, 52–53, 129
    as winner under national health insurance, 144
Mental Health Parity and Addiction Act of 2008 (MHPAA), 52
Mifepristone, 85
Milbank, Dana, 139
Milliman Medical Index (2018), 130
Money and politics
    corporate contributions to federal elections, 7–9, 7f
    stock buybacks and corporate profits, 8
    who Congress listens to, 8f
Moyers, Bill, 111
Mulvaney, Mick, 96
Musk, Elon
    America PAC, 8
    as "co-president" under Trump, 108
    leading Department of Government Efficiency, 9, 108–109
    X as political platform for, 7–8
Mystal, Elie, 83, 88

N

Nader, Ralph
    on health care fraud, 98–99
    on Medicare Advantage practices, 48
    justice and civic action, 136
Nation on the Take: How Big Money Corrupts Our Democracy and What We
    Can Do About It (Potter and Penniman), 31
National health insurance (NHI)
    building political support for, 147
    health care affordability and, 120
    losers under, 144–145, 145t
    McCanne on necessity for, 142
    Nixon's "Pay or Play" proposal, 2
    as solution for health care fraud, 99
    Theodore Roosevelt on, 2
    transition period from fee-based services, 153
    transition period from for-profit systems, 145

Truman's proposal (1946), 2
Trump on, 1
Trumpcare vs., winners and losers, 142–143
winners under, 143–144, 145t
National Registry of Evidence-Based Programs and Practices (NREPP), 52
Noah, Timothy, 140
Nursing homes
deregulation of, 104–105
for-profit profiteering, 30
fraudulent billing practices, 98
safety and accountability problems, 117

O

Obama, Barack, 3
Office of National Drug Control Policy, 115
Opioids, 114–115
Outcome of care, national health insurance and, 143
Out-of-network care, mental health, 52

P

Page, Benjamin, and Gilens, Martin, Democracy in America? What Has Gone
Wrong and What Can We Do About It, 34
Patient protections, loss of
deterioration of health safety net, 66, 134–136
employer-sponsored insurance, 66
exclusion of essential health benefits, 62–63
impacts of, 63–66
Medicaid eligibility requirements, 63
Medicare and Medicaid, 64, 65f
network restrictions and loss of choice, 65
pre-existing conditions, 60–61
premium increases for ACA coverage, 62
unaffordable premiums under ACA, 64
uninsured and underinsured, increases in, 65
women's health care and, 64
Patient protections, national health insurance and, 143
Penniman, Nick, 31
Pharmaceutical industry

avoidance of controls, 114

corporate greed trumping patient safety, 104

former congressional staffers working for, 28

lax regulatory practices, 103–104

Pfizer donations to Trump's inauguration, 28

price gouging, 29–30, 114, 127

Pharmaceutical Research and Manufacturers of America (PhRMA), lobbying by, 27–28, 29

Pharmacy-benefit managers, and drug price increases, 32

Physicians

burnout, 92

as winners under national health insurance, 144

Physicians and administrators, increase in, 1970–2019, 5f

Potter, Wendell, 20, 113

Potter, Wendell and Penniman, Nick, Nation on the TakeTake: How Big Money Corrupts Our Democracy and What We Can Do About It, 31

Pre-authorization of services, 136

Pre-existing conditions

denial of coverage, 60–61, 60f

Trump on, 59

Presidential election (2024), voter results on abortion policy and reproductive rights, 87–88

Price, Tom, 21, 96

Prior authorizations, time required for, 93

Prisons

mental illness and incarceration, 117

privatized, 52–53, 117

The Privatization of Everything: How the Plunder of Public Goods Transformed America and How We Can Fight Back (Cohen and Mikaelien), 43

Privatization of health care

as corporate welfare, 16

extent in U.S., 45–53

for-profit ownership, 2016, 46f

health care efficiency myth, 12

historical perspective, 42–44

maximization of profits, 55, 126

Medicaid, 30, 48, 90

Medicare, 46–49

mental health care, 52–53

myth of private sector efficiency, 43

negative impacts of, 44

private insurers as losers under national health insurance, 144–145

private Medicare and Medicaid enrollments, 45

social health insurance vs., 54

Veterans Administration, 50

Profit centers, diagnoses as, 126

Profiteering, upcoding and, 92–93

Project 2025 Mandate for Leadership: The Conservative Promise (Heritage Foundation), 78–79, 126

Pruitt, Scott, 118

Public health

as winner under national health insurance, 144

Q

Quality of care

inadequecies, 131–132

national health insurance and, 143

R

Rannazaisi, Joe, 114

Redford, Robert, 118

Reich, Robert

on common good, 123

on re-election of Trump, 25

Relman, Arnold S., 14–15, 125

Reproductive rights

medication abortion, 85

Supreme Court striking down Roe v. Wade ruling (2022), 83–84

in vitro services and fetal personhood, 85

Roosevelt, Franklin D., 27

Roosevelt, Theodore, 2

S

Sanders, Bernie, 142–143

Seniors. See Elderly persons

Single payor insurance. See National health insurance (NHI)

SNAP (Supplemental Nutrition Assistance Program), 134

Social Insurance: America's Neglected Heritage and Contested Future (Marmor, Mashaw, and Pakutka), 55

Sparrow, Malcolm, 97

Starr, Paul, 13–14

Stiglitz, Joseph, 45

Stock buybacks, corporate greed and, 8

Supplemental Nutrition Assistance Program (SNAP), 134

Supreme Court, striking down Roe v. Wade ruling (2022), 83–84

Surgery centers, regulatrory needs for, 103

T

Tax Equity and Fiscal Responsibility Act (TEFRA), 44

Taxpayers, as winner under national health insurance, 144

Truman, Harry S., national health insurance proposal (1946), 2

Trump, Donald

    alliance with Musk, 9

    conflicts of interest in first term, 94

    dictatorship ambitions, 123

    health care politics in turmoil, 146

    on health insurance for all (2017), 1

    minimizing government role in health care regulation, 139

    reduction of prescription drug prices as priority (2017), 30

    short-term health insurance proposals, limitations of, 115

    toxic ethical standards of first term, 96

    warnings about second term, 36–37

Trumpocracy: The Corruption of the American Republic (Frum), 22

21st Century Cures Act, lowering approval standards for new drugs, 104

U

Under-insured population

    bare-bone policies and, 128

    barriers to affordable health care, 71

Uninsured population, barriers to affordable health care, 70–71, 128

V

Verma, Seema, 4

Veterans Administration (VA)

attempts to privatize, 50–51

quality of care vs. non-VA hospitals, 51f

W

Weissman, Robert, 95

Welfare opposition, increase in, 135–136

Who Rules the World? (Chomsky), 22

Women's health care

cuts to Medicaid and, 136

loss of patient protections and, 66, 128–129

About the Author

John Geyman, M.D. is professor emeritus of family medicine at the University of Washington School of Medicine in Seattle, where he served as Chair of the Department of Family Medicine from 1976 to 1990. As a family physician with over 21 years in academic medicine, he also practiced in rural communities for 13 years. He was the founding editor of *The Journal of Family Practice* (1973 to 1990) and the editor of *The Journal of the American Board of Family Medicine* from 1990 to 2003. Since 1990 he has been involved with research and writing on health policy and health care reform.More recently, he has shifted his interest to national politics, the increasing polarization across our country, and their imminent threat to American democracy.

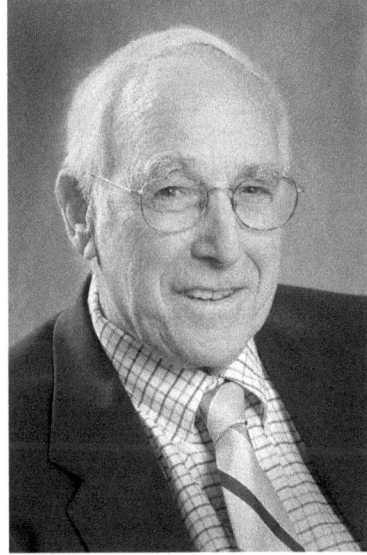

His most recent book is *Corporate Power and Oligarchy, How Our Democracy Can Prevail Over Authoritarianism and Fascism* (2024), *Are We the United States of America, Can We Hold Together as One Country?* (2022), *The Future of U.S. Health Care: Corporate Power vs. the Common Good*, (2022), *Transformation of U.S. Health Care, 1960-2020: One Family Physician's Journey* (2022), *America's Mighty Medical-Industrial Complex: Negative Impacts and Positive Solutions* (2021), *Profiteering, Corruption and Fraud in U.S. Health Care* (2020), *Long Term Care In America: The Crisis All Of Us Will Face In Our Lifetimes* (2020), *Struggling and Dying Under Trumpcare* (2019), *TrumpCare: Lies, Broken Promises, How It Is Failing, and What Should Be Done?* (2018), *Crisis in U.S. Health Care: Corporate Power vs. the Common Good* (2017), *The Human Face of ObamaCare: Promises vs. Reality and What Comes Next* (2016), *How Obamacare Is Unsustainable: Why We Need a Single-Payer Solution For All Americans* (2015), *Souls on a Walk: An Enduring*

Love Story Unbroken by Alzheimer's (2013), *Health Care Wars: How Market Ideology and Corporate Power Are Killing Americans* (2012), *Breaking Point: How the Primary Care Crisis Threatens the Lives of Americans* (2011), *Hijacked: The Road to Single Payer in the Aftermath of Stolen Health Care Reform* (2010), *The Cancer Generation: Baby Boomers Facing a Perfect Storm* (2009), *Do Not Resuscitate: Why the Health Insurance Industry Is Dying* (2008), *The Corrosion of Medicine: Can the Profession Reclaim Its Moral Legacy* (2008), *Shredding the Social Contract: The Privatization of Medicare* (2006), *Falling Through the Safety Net: Americans Without Health Insurance* (2005), *The Corporate Transformation of Health Care: Can the Public Interest Still Be Served?* (2004), *Health Care in America: Can Our Ailing System Be Healed?* (2002), *Family Practice: Foundation of Changing Health Care* (1985), and *The Modern Family Doctor and Changing Medical Practice* (1971).

John has also published five pamphlets following the approach of Thomas Paine in 1775-1776: *Common Sense About Health Care Reform in America* (2017), *Common Sense: U.S. Health Care at a Crossroads in the 2018 Congress* (2018), *Common Sense: The Case For and Against Medicare For All. Leading Issue in the 2020 Elections* (2019), *Common Sense: Medicare For All: Foundation for a 'New Normal' In U.S. Health Care* (2020), and *Common Sense: Medicare For All: What Will It Mean For Me?* (2021), and *U.S. Health Care at a Crossroads: Is it finally time for National Health Insurance?* (2025)

He also served as the president of Physicians for a National Health Program from 2005 to 2007, and is a member of the National Academy of Medicine.

Order additional copies of this book, *Growing Costs of U.S. Health Care Corporate Power vs. Human Rights: Is it Finally Time For Real Change?* from Amazon.com ($21.95) or as a Kindle eBook ($5.99).

Copies of the *Common Sense* pamphlet can also be ordered from Amazon.com for $5.95, or as a Kindle eBook version ($2.99).

www.ingramcontent.com/pod-product-compliance
Lightning Source LLC
Chambersburg PA
CBHW040855210326
41597CB00029B/4851